Bonding
with
Nature

Design by Claire MacMaster, barefoot art graphic design

Printed by Printworks Global Ltd. London & Hong Kong
First Edition

ISBN 13: 978-0-9973920-9-8

Bonding
with
Nature

Responding to Life's Challenges
and the Aging Process

The Transformational Power of Our National Parks,
Community Preserves, and Your Own Backyard

Dianna K. Emory

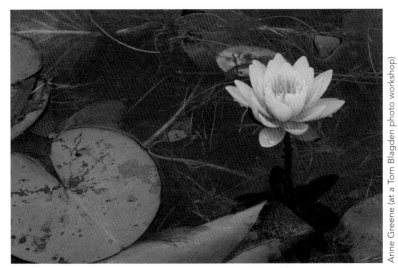

The Promise of Life.

Anne Greene (at a Tom Blagden photo workshop)

INTRODUCTION

What ever-present resource can relax and energize us, restore positive feelings, feed and strengthen our bodies, provide companionship, and help us to move more comfortably through challenging times? Our natural world is available at no cost whenever we want to access it—whether in our home environment, around our communities, or in one of a plethora of protected spaces, from local land trusts to national parks. When immersion in nature and a connection to living things are teamed up with a healthy diet, visualization techniques, regular exercise, volunteerism, and other strategies, the result is a winning combination that will see us through the most challenging times of our lives and carry us through old age.

As I turned to the natural world to help me navigate through childhood cancer and later the responsibilities of adult life, I also steered toward advanced degrees in the mental health field that armed me with cognitive-behavioral strategies to address the mental and physical needs of my patients. Personally challenging medical encounters had silver linings that helped me to better understand how to most effectively guide others to care for their bodies, their minds, and the world around them.

A long history of volunteerism in environmental organizations equipped me to assist others in learning about opportunities where they could impact the health of the natural world, while helping themselves as well. An increasing awareness of the fragility of life and a reconfirmation that we must grasp every moment propelled me forward. Deep engagement in our protected lands and green spaces through athletic and spiritual endeavors prepared me to enthusiastically encourage others to follow that path. Weaving in all sorts of activities that strengthen our connection with the natural environment, from gardening to bird watching, helped to build a treasure chest of other resources. And, the understanding that we can take our recreational and sensory experiences and translate them into memories that we store for future use brought me to the transformational power of our parks, preserves, and the natural world: making it last a lifetime.

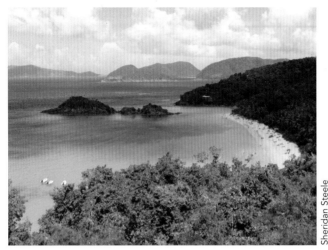

Trunk Bay, St. John, VINP: with Help, the Natural World Can Recover.

A POST-HURRICANE TRIBUTE TO VIRGIN ISLANDS NATIONAL PARK

Hurricane Irma's extraordinary power devastated Virgin Islands National Park, St. John, and many other Caribbean islands just as this book was being completed. The natural world is resilient and has recovered from many traumas since Earth's creation. It can happen this time, too. I pray that such a strong hurricane is an anomaly, although I believe the contradicting evidence offered by climate change experts. I wish that the people and the creatures in Irma's path could heal as rapidly as the tropic vegetation, but it is not that simple. My husband, Ben, and I reeled as we read of the destruction and contemplated the long healing process ahead for this beloved part of the natural world and its people.

Despite a firm belief in the impact of human activity on climate change, I am guilty of trusting that in the short-term, at least, we can count on the natural world to be a place to which we can turn as long as our bodies allow it. For most of my adult life, I have been wedded to

4

Virgin Islands National Park, its flora and its fauna. I assumed that my health or my vision would eventually give out but that, for now, I could count on returning to that magnificent part of the world for physical activity, emotional connection, and spiritual renewal. It did not occur to me that the entire island chain, of which St. John is a part, could be so drastically affected so quickly and that the natural world and its people would likely not be the same in my lifetime. As a tribute to the Park, I have kept things in this book as they were before the hurricane, with the hope that we can help it to recover.

Joe Kessler, President of Friends of Virgin Islands National Park and a treasured friend, tells me that two recovery funds have been established: Friends of St. John Recovery Fund, which is directed to local social service organizations working on relief and recovery, and Virgin Islands National Park Recovery Fund, which supports Park recovery efforts. All author royalties from this book through 2019 will be directed to these funds. After that time, they will go to medical institutions and organizations working on behalf of the natural world and her creatures.

1

OUR HISTORIES SHAPE OUR CONNECTIONS TO THE NATURAL WORLD

"Look deep into nature
and you will understand everything better."
Albert Einstein

If you picked up this book, you could have written it. You likely already feel a deep connection to the natural world—whether in your own backyard, a protected green space, or one of our national, state, or community parks—a passion we share. We want our time in those places to go on and on. We often seek them out for just plain fun, but there are other reasons as well. Memories of romping with pets across sweet-smelling fields, launching bugs on matchstick rafts, diving deep into bracing waters, trekking with family through snow-laden woods, mucking about in marshes scooping up tadpoles and newts, and perching in treetops surreptitiously to gaze down at the world below—these are a part of our spirit. We want to share those experiences with our loved ones and the next generation, hoping that they will be stimulated to seek the same and, one day, take on our roles as stewards of this threatened world. We mentor our message in many ways. We rise at dawn to squeeze in a brain-stimulating bike ride, run, or cross-country ski, knowing that we will be sharpened for a day of intellectual challenges. We feel deeply that we need those endorphin-releasing experiences and other connections to the natural world to be at our best. We seek out paintings, gardens, music, literature, and other artistic connections to our environment and, in many cases, try our own hand at depicting nature. And, we quietly contemplate remarkable vistas, rejoicing at each new day, while praying for the strength to make it through a difficult period as we are pushed through the challenge. We may reflect on all of this and ponder how we got to this place in life, how we can stay engaged in the things that we value, and how we can make a difference to the world.

This book encourages you to engage deeply with the environment—employing your passions to enhance daily life and build a reservoir for times when active use of the natural world is not available. As you tap your own life-enriching inner resources, you can care for yourself, other people, and the environment in a highly productive manner. Cognitively and behaviorally, you can be the facilitator of change as you learn to use your creativity to build strong visual, auditory, tactile, and olfactory memories of your engagement with the environment. And, when life puts up a roadblock, you can access this reservoir and incorporate it into powerful visualizations while also employing a wide variety of other experiences that are connected to the natural world. Reaching toward our parks and green spaces, drawing upon your own knowledge and the wisdom of others, you can impact your quality of life—even during overwhelming times.

You can take an approach that may be new to you, like visualization, combine it with things you know well, like a healthy diet and regular exercise, integrate your passions—from painting to caring for pets—and employ the natural world and her creatures as the forces that bind everything together. Regardless of life circumstances, through partnering with nature we can move forward one step at a time.

Early life experiences and treasured family members inspired my commitment to the natural environment and green space activities. Several sections in this book will illustrate how the silver linings in the clouds took me to a better place.

As a childhood cancer survivor with a bad case of post-traumatic stress disorder, my good fortune came in a life-saving connection to two environmental stewards. My grandmother, an early advocate for the intersection of art and nature, and my uncle, a research biologist, devoted themselves to my recovery. The threat of early death tormented me. Engagements with nature got me through the difficult periods, healed my body and my spirit, and saw me on to the time when I could keep up with everyone else.

Emotional and physical pains were soothed through expeditions into the woods, fields, and along the shorelines. The healing waters of Sebago Lake and the Atlantic Ocean transported me to a happier place. My favorite contacts were the bugs and the birds, the amphibians and the fish, and the many mammals that befriended me. My grandmother helped me create replicas of these beloved creatures through the paints and clay that were her tools. She, my parents, and my uncles took me out into nature at every turn and passed on their own knowledge and love of green spaces. When I was really struggling, I found that I could employ my commitment to the environment in creative ways until the next time that I could immerse myself in its lands and waters. These experiences were coupled with early spiritual messages and a strong survival instinct.

Who and what in your own history inspired you to develop a passionate environmental connection? Now would be a good time to begin a journal, make some notes, record some thoughts, or talk with others about this topic. You will likely find that some memories surface that you haven't thought about in years. As I write these words, I am smiling at my own recollections and hope that the same may be happening for you. Even those who are no longer in this world leave so much of themselves with us, don't they? Right now, facial images might come into your mind of loved ones who have left this world. Just enjoy those faces and the memories for a moment before we move on.

Perhaps you will identify with some of the following resounding messages that surface from my memory bank or maybe they will encourage you to recall some of your own. My recurring mantra is a passage from the Twenty-third Psalm that underscores the healing potential of the natural world. "He maketh me to lie down in green pastures. He leadeth me beside the still waters. He restoreth my soul." The depth of our need for green spaces and nature is powerfully conveyed in this universal message. Regardless of our religious orientation, we who are committed to the environment absorb this spiritual message with understanding. These words ring true for us and remind us to seek out the natural world in a multitude of ways so that we will be healthy, happy, and fulfilled for as long as possible. When activity, fitness, and immersion in nature are readily available to us, we bounce out the door with our dog, climb a mountain, jump on a bike, steam off on our cross-country skis, or gallop our horse down a gravel road. We release our endorphins, get a natural high, and fill ourselves with the beauty of the natural world and her creatures. Likewise, we portray nature through every art form, volunteer on behalf of its preservation, rejoice with others on its merits, and reach toward it for inner peace and renewal.

A large body of research[14, 54, 76, 77, 85, 86, 87, 88] confirms the fact that we *need* exposure to nature. It fills our senses as we breathe deeply of the scents of springtime, watch the soaring of a bird across the sky, are mesmerized by the bubbling of a spring, or are awe-struck by the crash of surf upon a craggy shore. When we are unable to engage with the green world, we know that something very important is missing. We may feel stressed, anxious, depressed, and deprived of an element that is crucial to our health. Medical professionals and scientists tell of the vital connection between fitness and wellness, the merits of outdoor exercise over indoor activities, and the negative impact of being "plugged in," indoors, and away from nature. From our own personal experiences, scientists or not, we know they are correct.

The challenge comes in how to continue to connect with our soul and body-nurturing environment, and provide ourselves with an over-arching healthy lifestyle, now and when we are overwhelmed by work and responsibilities, halted by medical challenges, or slowed down by the effects of aging. One answer can be found in learning to derive daily inspiration and stimulation in new ways, preserving our active experiences in nature to use later when life is more constrained. Each of us has a host of memories of experiences in the natural world, as well as the ability to tap into our inner resources and tune in to all aspects of our innermost selves in order to achieve our wellness goals. I have done this many times over—for myself, for my clinical counseling patients, for those facing traumatic illness, for friends and family, and for professional peers. Let's reflect on our histories and an experience outdoors. Then, let's think about how we can preserve those things to carry us through periods when we have no extra time, are slowed down due to illness or an accident, or are very elderly. As you read my thoughts about this, you can keep your journal handy and generate some of your own ideas along the way.

As an active athlete who has also experienced numerous medical and personal challenges, I know well how important it is to stay connected to the natural world. Each dawn as I head out the door for a run, paddle board, bike, swim, hike, or ski in either Acadia National Park, Virgin Islands National Park, or some other green space, thanks pour forth for my life in these marvelous places. And, during difficult periods when physical activity is limited, I have gotten outside as much as possible while also choosing alternative activities and visualizing my endeavors in the natural world in order to impact my physical and emotional condition. Actively engaging in extraordinary green spaces with nature's creatures at every turn is a great gift, particularly given the fact that, from early childhood through young adulthood, I did not think I would make it to the next birthday. The ability to store memories of these endeavors for later use is another gift to which you have access as well.

During my early years, I fought off the terror of visits to Boston Children's Hospital by climbing trees, interacting with all sorts of living creatures from bugs to bunnies, swimming in my beloved Sebago Lake, and, at night, immersing in the recalled thrill of galloping a horse up Canter Hill or swimming through ocean eelgrass. The loss of my 41-year-old father to cancer when I was 17 led me to pursue endorphin-releasing bike rides and quiet meditations focused on times shared with him in a pristine lake and woods—activities that helped me paw through my depression. Several more surgeries as a young, then aging, adult offered opportunities to employ the same creative visualization and guided imagery I used with my patients who were suffering from the effects of multiple sclerosis, cancer, or mental health issues—techniques in which I had doctoral-level training and that I had also unwittingly employed to my own advantage since childhood. When stage three breast cancer struck my young daughter, Melissa, we both pulled out all the stops—exercising vigorously in our parks and other green spaces, impacting positive change for ourselves and others where we could, and using every cognitive-behavioral technique we knew in order to make it through each day. Like me, Melissa was steeped in alternative healing techniques that she now uses with her own patients.

Beyond active engagement outdoors, one of the most helpful things I found during Melissa's illness was the constant reminder of remarkable experiences in beloved places and those who had shared those experiences. Deep relationships with friends and family whom I could now watch moving through easier times, and whose joy I could share, helped immensely. Asked repeatedly by friends how they could assist, I responded, "Tell me of the good things in your life and the high points of your days. That is uplifting."

My volunteer work on behalf of the lands and waters went on a parallel track to feed my spirit each day. Volunteerism bolstered my own recovery during a series of life crises. Leadership roles in the fund-raising and land protection efforts of Friends of Acadia and Maine Coast Heritage Trust were places where I could make a difference during a time when I felt that Melissa's recovery from cancer was beyond my control.

BUILD A MEMORY BANK

You don't need a history of personal or familial traumatic illness to derive great benefit from immersion in the natural world. All you need are normal developmental events and the desire and the determination to bring the environment into your life on a regular basis—through outdoor activities or substitutes for those engagements when they are not available. Your inspiration and passion for the green outdoors could come from athletic activities, moments of solitude, connections with birds and other creatures, scientific curiosity, the arts, or the anticipation of what is over the next mountain. For most of us, it is a combination of these and many other factors that weds us to the environment and makes us yearn for its beauty and restorative qualities. It stimulates us to weave the threads of past and present interaction with green spaces throughout our existence and prepares us to store those experiences in our sensory memory bank.

To build your memory bank, you can use the prepared scripts from this book as a model. Vividly recalling your own sensory experiences and learning to use them as a break during a busy day, or when you need some assistance during a crisis, are within easy reach. We will look at that in detail in Chapter Three. This technique is one thread of a tapestry of approaches that will help to build coping skills and the route to a healthier life. Here is an example of a memorable experience that helped me during Melissa's illness and to which I drift at times when active engagement in the natural world is interrupted due to work, responsibilities, or medical surprises.

Out of the Virgin Islands National Park darkness, bird songs stir—first quietly then robustly—welcoming the emerging dawn. The tropic's time of avian activity is before first light, as many songsters return to silence in the full heat of midday. When light allows, two kingfishers dart visibly in a courting dance, calling out their love. Their crested caps and blue highlights waltz along the coral shore. Could this pair have travelled thousands of miles to Acadia to grace the shores of the Schoodic District's Mill Stream last summer? If that is true, who are we to speak of our own limitations rather than rejoice in our potential? We reflect on the miracle of bird migration and the millions that make this yearly trek from Maine to the Eastern Caribbean and other remote places, as the murmur of other birds erupts from amidst the earthy vegetation.

Hummingbirds also abound along tropic shores, hovering over blooms of sage, coral vine, and hibiscus to refuel upon their nectar. Likewise, across Acadia, the ruby-throated hummingbirds gather up to do the same. Gently lifting him from the slate one summer day, I examine a tiny bird's iridescent feathers and pointed beak between his deadened eyes. Tears spill at this life snuffed out—he persevered o'er many miles to reach this summer place. Settling down to rest against the warm south-facing wall, I hold the little bird as tears streak down my cheeks. Is that movement in his twisted foot? It is. Then more. Forty minutes pass, as gradually the bird reclaims his life. He bobs uncertainly in my palm, takes flight, and shoots away. Twenty minutes more I sit, contemplating existence and wondering just how strong that little bird could be. A small, dark, and whirring dot zooms closer in to hover near. My hand welcomes back the tiny bird who comes to rest once more. He sits for seconds and, with determination, presses his sharp little beak into my palm, gives a hummingbird kiss of thanks, then speeds away. This much I know is true.

Each time I reflect on that passage, I am so thankful to be in this life with so many incredible creatures. That hummingbird vision always brings a smile. Now, let an image form of your own memorable outdoor experience. Close your eyes and go deep into the details of that experience, breathing freely and easily as you relax into those memories. See the shapes and colors, feel the textures, hear the sounds, inhale the scents, experience the tastes, and examine the details. In a few minutes, open your eyes and reflect on how you feel. You can refine and expand this technique to assist you immensely in all aspects of your life, from reduction of anesthesia during surgery and lowered blood pressure to greater life satisfaction and increased energy. It is an important beginning in a multi-faceted approach to engaging more deeply with the natural world. You might want to transfer your imagery into written form, embellishing the details and enriching the text. Then, you can use it on its own or combine it with one of the relaxation approaches included in Chapter Three.

We are remarkably fortunate to be in this place, in this world, in this time. How we landed here instead of in a more difficult place is a mystery but, as William Blake so aptly put it, "Every night and every morn, some to misery are born. Every morn and every night, some are born to sweet delight." Regardless of the extent of our own life challenges, or the depths of our miseries, most of us remain very, very fortunate and are blessed with "sweet delight" when compared to those who exist in much of the world. How do we take this good fortune and use it to assist the world while bettering ourselves physically, psychologically, and spiritually? And, how can we store it up for future use? Some of the answer lies in the way in which we use the natural treasures that have been bestowed upon us.

As a part of the route to feeling stronger emotionally, physically, and spiritually throughout the peaks and valleys of life, we will look at some conservation gems and how you can engage with them. We will also consider how you can augment what these places offer during periods when you cannot be active; how you can care for your body and your mind in a healthy manner; how you can connect more deeply with others in mutually beneficial relationships; how you can reach

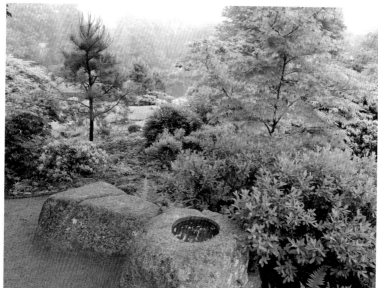

Asticou Azalea Garden: a Healing Place.

beyond yourself to give back for what you are given; and how to address each aspect of the natural environment and its creatures to maximize the benefit that can be derived on their and your own behalf. We will also delve into the world and the creatures of two outstanding ocean-oriented parks, Maine's Acadia National Park and Virgin Islands National Park, as models for engagement in any green space, including your own backyard or the green spaces within your home.

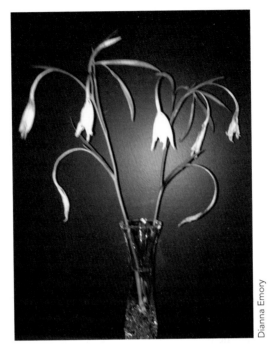

Stages of Life.

Dianna Emory

2

THE FIVE V'S TO MAKING THE TRANSFORMATIONAL POWER OF NATURE LAST A LIFETIME

"And allow the circumstances that present themselves to nudge you in the direction of the highest possible good."
Rasha from *Oneness*

When active engagement with the natural world and its creatures is limited, there are many possibilities that will continue to fill us with the joy of our green environment and all living things. As we engage with the world and her creatures, we can etch their details into our memories so that they can be retrieved at a later date to help us out. We will explore some of those options as well.

Visualizing enables us to bring green space experiences into our minds whenever we desire through tapping our memories and imaginations. This book helps you learn relaxation techniques and visualization approaches. It also provides relaxation therapy scripts, green space visualizations, and deepening methods for your adaptation and use. Texts and recordings based upon your own experiences or the use of those in this book can help to transport you through difficult periods—offering restoration, insight, relief, and hope for the future. Further assistance with these techniques can be found on my website, www.DiannaEmory.com.

Vetting means investigating various techniques to see which ones can help us the most. An investment in healthy habits will produce a solid return. Provided are charts and information related to exercise; healthy dietary choices; building support networks; choosing alternative or enrichment activities that complement the green outdoor experience; and employing relaxation and visual imagery techniques. These are for use now and during the times when we are slowed down by responsibilities, medical issues, or the aging process. These techniques will help to keep us strong, optimistic, and able to face life's challenges in a resilient manner. We can take all of these approaches and combine them with our interests in the natural world and her creatures so that we can maximize the benefits from our experiences.

Viewing other people's successes during difficult periods in their lives helps us to understand how we can cope with our own challenges. Case studies of people impacted by illness, stressors, and aging are provided, as are diaries and recollections from my own life as a mental health professional and conference presenter, survivor of a rare childhood cancer, and parent of a young adult impacted by traumatic illness.

Volunteering and making a commitment to assist an important cause takes us outside ourselves to employ our passions and our expertise as we act in the interest of others and the environment. If we do even one small thing each day to help another living thing or the world, we can feel that we are having some positive impact—even when our own situations might seem overwhelming. This book describes the benefits of volunteerism on behalf of various causes, including our national parks, land trusts, other conserved spaces, and the creatures that inhabit these places.

We can apply the Visualizing, Vetting, Viewing, Venturing Forth, and Volunteering framework to any green space that is available. As examples of how you can maximize your engagement with the natural world, we are going to **venture forth** and delve deeply into our home environments, Acadia National Park, Virgin Islands National Park, and other natural areas, to examine the land, the skies, and the waters of those places, as well as the creatures and other living things that are found there. We can rejoice in all that is provided for our exploration, examination, and enjoyment; we can employ this natural world to assist us through all stages of life. As stewards of the world, we can offer back the best that we can give to help to protect these exquisite lands, waters, and living things.

We acknowledge that life challenges can interfere with our ability to take full advantage of that natural world. Challenges can come in the form of work and personal stressors, brushes with illness, or the aging process. Fabricated case studies, representative of the kind of work I have done, are provided. These describe experiences of others who have learned to weave their memories and experiences into **visualizations** to help them through tough periods, maintain health, or initiate change. Each person's period of crisis involved the **vetting** of opportunities to

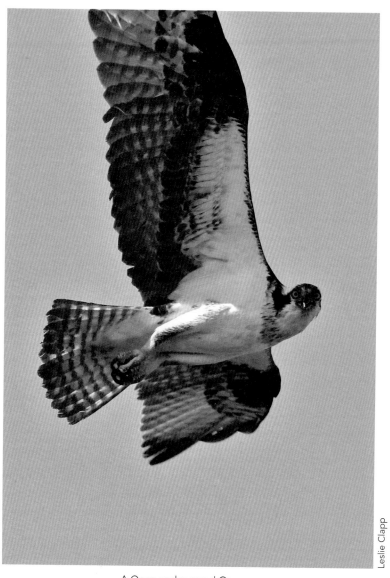

A Once-endangered Osprey.

Leslie Clapp

be in touch with the green outdoors as much as possible; vetting alternative activities to satisfy that need; vetting and choosing a healthy approach to diet and exercise; and vetting mutually beneficial relationships. **Volunteering** played a part for each person as well, as did **viewing** other people's routes to recovery. In Chapter 5, you can look at some examples of how others made it through the challenging periods. You can then move on to how you can engage with the natural world and use the Five V's effectively whenever you desire.

3

VISUALIZATION: CAPTURING YOUR MEMORIES AND EXPERIENCES

*"Look deep into nature and you will
understand everything better."*
Albert Einstein

Over forty years ago, when I first began using relaxation techniques and creative visualization in my clinical counseling practice, these methods were outside the realm of traditional medicine and mental health treatment. My unusual childhood experiences, from traumatic illness and surgery to the loss of a parent as a teen, led me to explore a host of ways to cope, as I describe in this book. Alternative approaches to healing came naturally to me and were integrated into my life in many ways. A desire to assist patients with chronic pain, surgical issues, major medical crises, anxiety, and depression was the inspiration to pursue formal training in these techniques and clinical hypnosis through the American Society of Clinical Hypnosis and its affiliates while simultaneously working on my master's degree and then my doctorate. In the 1970s and early '80s, my professional peers were physicians, dentists, and a handful of mental health practitioners. By 2007, membership in the American Society of Clinical Hypnosis had grown to over 2,000 from a small group in 1975. Rather than being fringe specialties, creative visualization, relaxation techniques, and clinical hypnosis had gone mainstream. Now, four decades of sound, scientific research have proved the positive impact that these techniques can have on the body and the mind. By 1987, clinical hypnosis and other relaxation approaches had been formally recognized as legitimate treatment modalities by the American Medical Association, the World Federation of Mental Health, the American Psychological Association, and the American Association for the Advancement of Science. Scores of research studies have documented their effectiveness.[4]

We are going to begin by keeping it simple. You can do these exercises on your own or with someone else. You can even record them or have someone read them to you, if you want.

Start by taking five deep breaths and having a big yawn and stretch, even if it feels contrived. Actually, it probably feels pretty good, doesn't it?

Now, close your eyes, breathing freely and deeply. Picture yourself in some relaxing place from your memory or your imagination. Fill your senses with that place—see the shapes, hear the sounds, see the colors, enjoy the tastes, smell the fragrances—put as much detail into the experience as you want, and just stay there for a few minutes. Then, open your eyes and think about how you are feeling. You just accomplished a visualization exercise. See how easy that is? Let's try it again. Was it even easier that time? You can practice visualizations any time you have a few minutes and want to relax. Imagine a peaceful, lovely place from your memory or imagination, incorporating all of the colors, scents, textures, and images you can. Go deep into each aspect of that place. You can refresh yourself easily and effortlessly, whenever you want.

The phrase "in your mind's eye"[93] is a great way to generate the visual image that you can get when picturing something in your mind. This happens all the time, with no effort. Images come easily and effortlessly when we focus on different thoughts. Some people are more visual than others, but we can all do this. Let your eyes drop closed again, take five deep breaths, and let yourself drift down, down to a more and more relaxed state. In your mind's eye get a picture of a pet or one of nature's other creatures you care about. Think about the details—the shapes, the sounds, the colors, the textures, the scents, and all the other sensory messages you get. Focus on the feelings you have when you are with that creature. You might want to think of a time you really enjoyed doing something with him or her. Just rest there for a few minutes and then open your eyes, feeling very, very good throughout.

Now, let's try a progressive body relaxation. Please find a comfortable place to recline where you will not be disturbed by telephones, pets, or other interruptions. Stretch out, without crossing your arms or legs, let your eyes drop closed, and begin breathing freely and deeply.

Focus on relaxation flowing in, tension flowing out, as you breathe freely and deeply and let everything go. Just put everything on hold and let yourself relax completely, breathing freely and deeply, freely and easily. As you relax more and more, imagine a warm, comfortable wave of relaxation flowing over your body. Start at the top of your head and move through each body part, focusing and letting each part go loose, limp, and relaxed as the warm, comfortable wave of relaxation flows over you. Rest in that comfortable condition as long as you want, knowing that your body is restoring itself physically, spiritually, and emotionally. Then open your eyes feeling completely refreshed, yet relaxed, with renewed energy.

(If you choose, use this technique to help you drift off into a deep, sound night's sleep rather than returning to alertness.)

You might want to try meditating, which is another form of deep relaxation. Choose a word or phrase upon which to focus. Sit upright, close your eyes, and focus your mind on your word or phrase. Breathe freely and deeply, relax your body, and repeat your word or phrase as you exhale. If your mind drifts away, nudge it gently back again. Continue for 15-20 minutes. What do you think of that? You might have already tried yoga's combination of stretching exercises, controlled breathing, and meditation—another very effective way of bringing on the relaxation response.

For another slant on things, get your pen and make a list of relaxing experiences. These might include hiking to a beautiful spot where you can put life in perspective, lying on the beach smelling the scent of the ocean, reading or cuddling your cat in your favorite chair, inhaling the scent of lavender, taking a warm bath, or sitting in a garden observing all that is around you. Give yourself the opportunity to re-visit some of these experiences and identify which ones bring you the greatest sense of calmness.

Now, we are ready for a very important tool. Reaching within our remarkable minds to engage our memories and our imaginations through creative visualization enables us to move to a comfortable space where we can refresh ourselves within minutes. We are rested and energized, our minds are clearer, and we move forward feeling much more positive. As caregivers for others, or in our professional duties, we are better prepared and we find things less overwhelming. As patients affected by accidents or illness, we move into surgery or the treatment process more easily and derive greater benefit. And, as aging adults, we easily access the experiences we hold dear while creating new adventures for the future. In each of these situations, the natural world and her creatures contribute heavily to the path to greater life satisfaction as we engage with them in whatever way we can, while also building a repertoire of details from which we can draw when we want to create meaningful visualizations.

During periods when we are overwhelmed with work or responsibilities, ill, injured, or just plain old, we may be unable to utilize all of the resources that normally help to keep us at peak wellness. That is the time that it is particularly important to engage in the relaxation response and creative visualizations from our memory or our imagination that can help us to feel so much better.

The included visualization and an accompanying download at www.DiannaEmory.com may be used to enhance physical and mental health and as a step beyond actual outdoor activity. Visualizations that can be integrated with relaxation approaches are sprinkled throughout this document in italics, and others are presented with the relaxation approaches in Chapter Three. These resources and the ones that you create can be used now and in the future when work, medical issues, family responsibilities, or old age interfere with your ability to get out and actively use your beloved green spaces.

Using these techniques can make a significant difference in each day and will add up to a life where everything comes a bit easier because stress has less opportunity to disrupt you. There has been an aura around visualization and relaxation approaches that has led people to think that they need someone else to "do it" to them. The fact is that these techniques are simple to learn and just require regular use for them to become very, very effective. Everything you do can be impacted—from managing your children in a calmer manner, to bringing down your level of irritation with a co-worker, to lessening the amount of anesthesia you need during surgery, to making a speedier recovery, to running faster, to bringing back the memories of expeditions into the green outdoors. That is quite a promise, isn't it? **The only requirement is that you never, never use a recording of these approaches when you are driving or operating machinery**. Case in point: over thirty years ago when I was doing a live recording of one of my tapes, the staff in the recording studio fell sound asleep (or into a deeply relaxed state) halfway through the recording. I had to shake them to wake them up! I have also watched dozens of people in large group relaxation sessions become so deeply relaxed that they have begun happily snoring away in unison—not the best situation for the non-snorers!

Now, I am going to type in a relaxation exercise for you that you can adapt in any way that you want to meet your needs. As I type the relaxing suggestions, I am going to try not to fall out of my chair in a state of loose, limp, and comfortable relaxation.

Relaxation and visualization scripts can be read to you or recorded for your use. Begin by reading scripts and changing details to meet your own needs, if you want. You will also find a download of one of my relaxation tapes available on my website, www.DiannaEmory.com. This recording targets increased energy, improved health, and general well-being and can be used by anyone who wants to use relaxation techniques as a part of a healthcare plan. Please read the instruction sheet. Absolutely DO NOT DRIVE OR OPERATE MACHINERY WHILE LISTENING TO ANY RELAXATION EXERCISE. You can fall asleep unexpectedly while hearing suggestions of relaxation.

Script: General Relaxation with Suggestions for Good Health

Start by getting yourself comfortable, sitting or lying down, without crossing your arms or legs. Let your eyes drop closed and begin breathing freely and deeply…freely and deeply…relaxing more and more with each breath… relaxation flowing in, tension flowing out. Relaxation flowing in…tension flowing out. Whatever happens for you is just fine. Just let yourself go…relaxing more and more with each breath. No worries, no cares need bother you now. This is your time to just put everything on hold and relax completely. No outside noises need disturb you. Instead, they will allow you to relax even more deeply, even more completely. Remember, you don't have to worry about performing correctly during this experience. However you respond is just fine. Your response may vary from one time to the next… sometimes you may drift in and out of awareness, hearing parts of what is said and seeming not to hear other parts. Other times you may follow along comfortably, feeling pleasantly relaxed. Or, you may drift off to what feels like a deep, sound sleep…awakening at the end of your session. Regardless of the manner in which you find yourself responding, you can derive significant benefits from this relaxing experience, even when you feel that you have slept throughout the session. All the positive messages help you to nurture your body and your mind—helping it to maintain good health or return to a very healthy condition.

If your attention drifts away, just nudge it gently back to the messages you are hearing, messages that help you to gain more control over your mind and your body and help you to strengthen yourself physically and emotionally. As you listen, you can become deeply relaxed, perhaps much more relaxed than you have been in a very long time. Like anything else, with practice you become even more adept at using relaxation techniques. Each time you relax even more deeply, even more completely.

Just let yourself go now, drifting freely and easily…freely and easily… down, down to a more and more comfortable place. No matter how deeply relaxed you go, if you need to alert yourself and give your attention to something else you can do so. Then, you can return to position and drift easily back down to a deeply relaxed condition, continuing with your relaxation session.

As you relax more and more, a warm comfortable wave of relaxation can begin to wash over your body, soothing and relaxing, soothing and relaxing…flowing over your scalp, soothing and penetrating, easing away all tension…flowing down over the sides and the back of your head, easing away all tension, relaxing completely, relaxing completely. The soothing wave of relaxation flows down over your face, easing away all tension… penetrating your forehead and brows…flowing over your eyes, giving them a warm, comfortable soothing bath that will give you clearer and sharper vision…relaxing completely…making you more and more comfortable, more and more relaxed. The wave of warm, comfortable relaxation flows down over your nose and cheeks, your mouth, your chin, and your jaw… letting everything go more and more relaxed…more and more limp and loose and relaxed…as the wave of relaxation flows down through your neck…penetrating the cords of your neck and head and face with so much relaxation that everything goes completely loose and limp and relaxed.

The wave of relaxation flows from your neck on down through your shoulders and upper arms, soothing and massaging, deep and relaxing, easing away all tension as you go more and more loose and limp and relaxed. The warm, comfortable wave of relaxation flows down through your elbows and forearms, easing away all tension…flowing down through your wrists, your hands, and your fingers…filling your arms and wrists, your hands and your fingers with so much relaxation that any remaining tension is pushed right out through the ends of your fingers…leaving everything feeling completely loose and limp and relaxed as you drift deeper and deeper into that warm, comfortable state of deep relaxation.

The warm, comfortable wave of relaxation flows from your neck down through your chest, soothing and penetrating, opening up your breathing passages so that with each breath clean, fresh air flows into your lungs, bringing with it a sensation of healing and wellness throughout. With each breath that you take, this soothing and healing energy flows into your body, continuing on even after you finish your session today…each breath, day and night effortlessly brings this healing energy into your body…and with it all of your body's inner resources are mobilized, assisting you in effortlessly strengthening everything about you…bringing your body and your mind to their healthiest possible condition. With each breath that you take, day and night…without even thinking about it…this sensation of strengthening and healing flows effortlessly into your body, bringing with it a feeling of wellness, deep relaxation, and comfort.

The wave of warm, comfortable relaxation flows from your chest and lungs down through your stomach, abdomen, and pelvis…soothing and relaxing, soothing and relaxing…easing away all tension, filling your stomach with a very pleasant and comfortable sensation…assisting your stomach in maintaining ongoing comfort throughout…assisting your body and your mind in choosing the foods and beverages that you know will help you to achieve and maintain your healthiest possible condition.

The warm, comfortable wave of relaxation rests again for a moment in the back of your neck...soothing and penetrating...deep and relaxing... massaging away all tension as it flows down into your upper back and shoulders, easing away all tension, massaging away all tension...as it flows down through your middle back and lower back, soothing and penetrating, deep and relaxing...easing away all tension...flowing down through your buttocks...relaxing completely, relaxing completely...filling your entire body with so much relaxation that everything goes completely loose and limp and relaxed...loose and limp and relaxed.

The warm, comfortable wave of relaxation flows on down through your thighs, soothing and penetrating, flowing down through your knees, your calves, your ankles, your feet, and your toes...filling your legs and ankles, your feet, and your toes with so much relaxation that any remaining tension is pushed right out through the ends of your toes, leaving everything feeling completely loose and limp and relaxed...loose and limp and relaxed.

With each breath that you take, you become more and more relaxed and comfortable...peaceful...in love with the world and its creatures... committed to doing all that you can to assist in some way...realizing that you are gaining more and more control over your own mind and your own body...that you are tapping all of your body's inner resources easily and effortlessly...unleashing your creativity so that it can work effectively and efficiently on behalf of yourself, the world, and her creatures...bringing your body and your mind to their healthiest possible condition.

There may be a pleasant sensation of warmth and comfort seeping throughout your hands and arms, your feet and your legs, filling your whole body as you go deeper and deeper relaxed. You are becoming more and more relaxed. You can sink deeper and deeper still into the warm, comfortable state of deep relaxation.

Now you can follow the numbers from one to ten, going more and more relaxed with each number. One...slipping easily into a more relaxed state. Two, at the count of ten, perhaps you are much more relaxed than you have been in a very long time. Three, breathing so easily, so freely... with each breath a feeling of relaxation and a comforting, healing sensation flows into your body...and this healing sensation continues on as each day passes, soothing, healing and strengthening your body. Four...healing and protecting, healing and protecting...Five...strengthening all of your body's resources to bring you to the strongest and healthiest condition... Six...Seven...No matter how deeply relaxed you go, all your positive messages drift way down deep to assist you in strengthening your own mind and your own body...assisting you in making the healthiest choices of foods and beverages, assisting you in incorporating activities in the green environment into your life as much as possible...assisting you in incorporating consistent healthy exercise and relaxation experiences into your life...assisting you in doing your part for the world and her creatures...Eight...so pleasantly relaxed and comfortable throughout, absorbing good health, relaxation, and wellness throughout...Nine...with your body and your mind experiencing a maximum feeling of comfort and healing throughout...Ten. Deeply relaxed, completely relaxed, in a very safe and comfortable place.

As you rest comfortably, your body and your mind experience great benefits. You may even get a sense or an image of a healing white light or energy that flows throughout your body, caring for and nurturing your body and your mind, strengthening and healing, deep and relaxing. This sensation can continue right on with you through each day and night with no effort on your part. You find that, as a part of each day, you engage in some way with the natural world and that you choose outdoor exercise as much as possible. A balanced, healthy diet and the regular use of relaxation techniques can provide benefits as well. As each day passes, you feel stronger and healthier, more and more positive throughout...both physically and emotionally.

Now, while you remain very deeply relaxed, feeling very comfortable, safe and calm throughout, you can take a pleasant journey through your memory or imagination. Whenever you choose to alter the imagery to make it more personally appealing, you can do so easily and effortlessly without disturbing your very relaxed condition. Your mind is an amazing thing and it can help you in so many ways to strengthen yourself. I am going to count from one to ten. As each number passes, you can drift peacefully through time and space to the top of a beautiful grassy knoll on a warm spring day. When I reach ten, you can be there in your mind's eye...on that beautifully grassy knoll on a warm spring day, feeling very, very good throughout... looking down over a sloping field of early spring flowers toward a peaceful pond below.

One...in your mind's eye you are drifting away from the present toward that grassy knoll. Two...by the time I reach ten, you can be there on the knoll, feeling so relaxed and pleasant throughout. Three...four... you are drifting closer and closer to the knoll. Whenever you choose to arrive there is just fine. Five...six...seven...You begin to see the details of the knoll as you get closer. You can see the vividness of the colors of the grass, the flowers, and the pond below. The sun can shine upon you with a comfortable level of intensity. Never burning, only comforting. You can spread a blanket upon the grass that will invite you to settle in. You inhale the fragrance of springtime and relax even more. Your sinuses remain clear and unaffected by any grasses or blossoming flowers. Eight...everything feels very, very good throughout. Nine...ten. There you are on the knoll, settling down comfortably with your blanket beneath you. No cares, no worries need bother you now. You can lie down comfortably and look up at the clear, blue sky above...feel the warmth of the sun upon your skin...never burning... always soothing. You can inhale deeply of the fragrance of springtime, letting your body fill with relaxation and peacefulness with each breath. Feel the joy of the moment...the delight in life...enjoying each moment to the fullest. No worries, no cares need bother you now. Let this feeling remain with you, breathing deeply and effortlessly, filling your mind and your body with joy, good health, peace, and relaxation throughout.

You feel so good as you lie there comfortably...you can reflect on all of the positive things in your life...how you can move past challenges to easier times...all of the people you care about, events from the past or the present that give you nice warm feelings... realizing how fortunate you are...deeply appreciating each aspect of your life. You can feel very, very good about yourself as a person, proud of all of your character strengths, optimistic about your ability to develop to your maximum potential.

You find that your thoughts can be especially clear, that your ability to recall past information is superb, and that your concentration ability is particularly sharp. All of these qualities can be even more a part of you as each day passes and you can feel better and better throughout, both emotionally and physically. You can find that you are generally more productive, optimistic, and that you appreciate each moment to the fullest feeling very, very good about your life and your future.

While you continue to relax comfortably on that grassy knoll, you can learn to reach this pleasant level of relaxation whenever you desire. This can be very easy for you and can produce very helpful results. Whenever you want to refresh yourself quickly and enhance your health, you find that all you need to do is to close your eyes, take three deep breaths, and think to yourself, "Deep relaxation." Then you drift right down to that deeply relaxed place where you are right now…or perhaps even deeper…and you rest there for as long as you want. If you choose, you can drift easily and effortlessly to some pleasant imagery from your memory or your imagination, to a place where you feel very deeply relaxed and comfortable, examining all the details of that place through your mind's eye…feeling, hearing, smelling, tasting, and seeing all the details of that special place…focusing in on whatever you choose and experiencing all aspects of that place even more deeply. You can also focus on aspects of your life that you want to strengthen related to healthy lifestyle habits or improved health.

Whenever you use this brief relaxation technique in the future, after you have rested as long as you want and are ready to return to a fully alert state, you can count slowly backwards from ten to one, bringing yourself gradually back to an alert condition. At the count of five, you open your eyes but you might not be fully alert. At the count of one you are completely alert…relaxed, yet refreshed, with renewed energy…feeling very, very good throughout, both physically and emotionally.

You can feel confident that you can use this technique whenever you want to bring on a deep relaxation response and wonderful imagery of very special places from your memory or your imagination. Now, you can move away from your instruction in this relaxation technique and let yourself drift back to the grassy knoll on that warm spring day. In your mind's eye, see how green and fresh the spring grasses are, how each blade springs up through the ground to greet the day. If you put your nose close to the ground, you can smell the sweetness of the grass and the earth. As you rest on the cushion of grass beneath your blanket, you can sink deeper into comfort and relaxation, feeling very, very good throughout. With each breath that you take, the fresh spring air can fill your lungs, soothing and healing, soothing and relaxing. You may get a sense or a feeling of the warm, gentle spring breeze caressing your relaxed body. You breathe freely and deeply, freely and easily. The sky is a deep, rich blue and the sun shines down upon you, always soothing, never burning. You may notice the call of a bird, the sound of the water lapping against the shore below, or the breeze blowing gently through the trees at the edge of the field. You can carefully examine all that is around you, making what you want of it, enjoying this special place as much as you choose.

Perhaps you will even get a sense, or a feeling, or an image in your mind's eye of a butterfly that has landed near you on a spring flower. Your eyes trace the gentle curve of the flower's stem up to its blossom where the butterfly perches. The flower can be any color or species that you want, as can the butterfly. Examine the intricate detail of the butterfly's wings, how her tiny legs hold the flower...the clear definition of the colors and designs on her wings...the slight movement as she rests there beside you. If you choose, you can invite her to climb gently upon your finger and sit there for a moment before you encourage her to lift herself into the air to fly to her next destination.

INSERT ANY OTHER SUGGESTIONS YOU CHOOSE HERE
(increased energy, positive feelings, speedy recovery from surgery, etc.)

For now, you can relax a bit longer on that grassy knoll, examining every detail. You are feeling very, very good throughout...focusing on the pleasant state you are in and feeling very comfortable in your ability to integrate relaxation techniques and positive imagery into your life. You can thoroughly experience what it is like to be there on that lovely knoll for a little while longer, inhaling the fragrance of springtime, letting each breath fill your body with good health and relaxation. Feel the warmth of the sun upon your body, always soothing, never burning. Hear the sound of a light breeze stirring the leaves upon the trees, the gentle lap of waves upon the shore of the pond below, the song of a bird in the distance. Experience the joy of the moment, the delight in life, and rest comfortably for a little while longer, realizing that you can return to this pleasant, relaxed state whenever you desire, and totally enjoying this wonderful condition of body and mind. And, remember, all of the benefits of deep relaxation and the suggestions for wellness that you have heard today continue right on with you even after we finish our session, strengthening and healing your body with each breath that you take.

In a few moments, as we count backwards from twenty to one, you can drift away from the grassy knoll and back to a fully alert state. At the count of one you will be fully alert and feeling very, very good throughout, both physically and emotionally, feeling as if you have just had a deep, refreshing night's sleep. You will feel proud of your ability to use relaxation techniques whenever you desire and realize that, with each experience similar to the one you used today, you will derive even greater benefits. You look forward to each new day and all that it can hold, finding yourself to be more productive and more satisfied in all that you do. You enjoy using your relaxation techniques on a daily basis, in concert with a healthy diet, regular exercise, and a deep and satisfying engagement with the world and her creatures.

Now, we begin to count backwards from twenty to one. With each number, you will come closer to a fully alert state. At the count of five, you will open your eyes, but you may not be completely alert. At the count of one, you will be completely alert, feeling relaxed, yet refreshed with renewed energy. You will have no stiffness, heaviness, numbness, or pain in any part of your body and will be feeling very, very good throughout, both physically and emotionally---relaxed, yet refreshed, with renewed energy.

Ready...20...starting to drift back through time and space...19...18... the scene on the grassy knoll is starting to fade, but you can return whenever you choose...17...16...15...by the time we reach the count of one you will have returned to your previous setting and will be completely alert, feeling very, very good throughout, much better than when we began this session...14...13...12...moving closer to alertness...11...10...9... at the count of 5 you open your eyes, but you might not be feeling completely alert...8...7...6...5...coming back from the grassy knoll to the present...4...3...2...1! Completely alert, refreshed, yet relaxed, with renewed energy...No pain, stiffness, heaviness, or numbness in any part of your body. Feeling very, very good throughout, both physically and emotionally. Looking forward to the rest of the day and evening, looking forward to each new day.

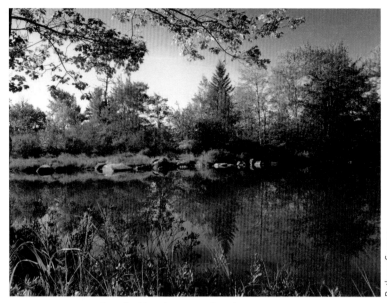

Bethany Savage

Ripe for Visualization: a Pond in Autumn.

You can add positive suggestions and additional visualization material to this script if you choose. Insert your material in the space indicated above.

There are so many routes to relaxation, visualization techniques, and a healthier lifestyle. The key is to find what works best for you and incorporate some of these techniques into your routine. The more you use any relaxation approach, the easier it is to derive benefits. Like anything else, practice will help.

4

VETTING: CHOOSING HEALTHY APPROACHES THAT WORK

"If we could give every individual the right amount
of nourishment and exercise, not too little and not too much,
we would have found the safest way to health."
Hippocrates, 460-377 BC

You now have the opportunity to vet and choose the engagements that can keep you going at full speed every day and/or help you if you are facing a challenge. Please don't worry about doing everything perfectly. You will find that this is all much easier than it seems on the surface. I confess that there have been chunks of time when I have not practiced what I preach. Sometimes I just run my butt off day after day, counting on the endorphins to keep me charging along in a positive direction, ignoring the need for sleep. Other times I use up every second of my day and think that the next day will give me more time to do all of the things I want to, including using relaxation approaches. Of course there is the evening when I grab the ice cream at the market and proceed to make us a big dessert. Some days, when the wind is howling and the temperatures have plunged, I stay at the computer all day, wishing it were summer. Then, I get back at it again and realize how much I have been missing—how much I can impact every step of my journey. You can do this for yourself as well. Just start now. Make a statement right out loud every morning and write it down as an affirmation. And, make it present, not future-oriented. *I get outdoors or engage with nature in the most active way that I can within the next several hours. I care for my body by feeding it well today. I integrate visualization and relaxation techniques into this day. I express thanks for today. I do at least one thing for the world and her creatures today. I reach out to friends and/or family today. I nurture and make my life space a little more beautiful today. I feel so good in this moment in time.*

All of our adventures in the natural world can be enhanced if we are taking as active a role as possible in caring for our bodies, our minds, and our relationships with the world and her creatures, while also creating nurturing spaces in which to live and play. The approaches we address through the vetting process can work collaboratively with every aspect of our engagement with the green outdoors. The natural world and her creatures can stand on their own and have huge impact on our lives, but they can do so much more for us when we are using them as a part of a package of healthy approaches to life.

As you know, the mind, body, and spirit each serve an important function in the maintenance of good health. Science has taught us that we can directly impact our well-being through using a multitude of easily accessible inner resources. These techniques can greatly impact the quality of our daily lives. In times of physical or emotional stress, tapping these tools can often make the difference between a speedy recovery and a struggle. Surgeries can be easier, depression can be lifted, pain can be lessened, and fatigue can be alleviated when we mobilize these resources and learn how to access the mind-body connection. Through making educated choices about the food and beverages that we put into our bodies; exercising regularly; maintaining a social network; doing good things for others; staying in touch with our spiritual selves; reaching toward activities that help to enrich our lives; giving back for what we have been given; and learning to use relaxation and visualization techniques, we can impact the way we are feeling each day. And, if the need arises, we are better-prepared to face physical or emotional crisis. One thing we know is, if we are lucky, we will continue to age and that process alone presents its challenges. We can prepare ourselves to be resilient.

During periods when we are overwhelmed with work or responsibilities, ill, injured, or just plain old, we may be unable to utilize all of the resources that normally help to keep us at peak wellness. That is the time that it is particularly important to engage in the relaxation response and creative visualizations from our memory or our imagination that can help us to feel so much better. These techniques can greatly enhance our quality of life through providing a well-rounded cognitive-behavioral approach to health care when they are combined with time outdoors engaging with the world and its creatures; activities to fill in for those things when we cannot get outside; a healthy diet and exercise plan; relationships with family and friends that create a mutual support system that encourages venting of emotions; and a commitment to give back for what we are given through volunteerism. There is never a better time than the present to employ the wealth of resources that are well-documented as having positive impact on our health.

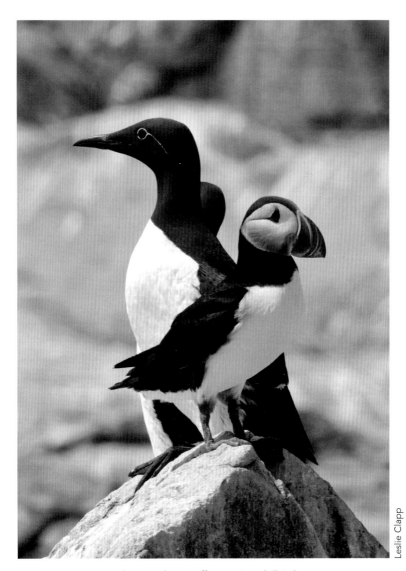

Find a Friend in a Puffin or a Razorbill Auk.

Leslie Clapp

BUILDING RELATIONSHIPS/MAINTAINING
A MUTUAL SUPPORT SYSTEM

*"Remember, spend some time with your loved ones, because they are not
going to be around forever. Remember, say a kind word to someone who
looks up to you in awe, because that little person soon will grow and leave
your side. Remember, to give a warm hug to the one next to you because that
is the only treasure you can give with your heart and it doesn't cost a cent.
Remember to say, "I love you" to your partner and your loved ones, but most
of all mean it. A kiss and an embrace will mend hurt when it comes from
deep inside of you. Remember to hold hands and cherish the moment,
for someday that person will not be there again. Give time to love, give time
to speak, and give time to share the precious thoughts in your mind."*
George Carlin, comedian, 2004

Asked by Thomas Friedman what is the biggest current disease in
America, Surgeon General Murphy replied, "It's not cancer. It's not
heart disease. It's isolation. It is the pronounced isolation that so many
people are experiencing that is the great pathology of our lives today."[5]
The strength, comfort, and joy that come from strong ties to family and
friends can make a huge difference to all that we experience. Reams of
research tell us that those with strong family ties live longer, that those
who have close sibling relationships have fewer symptoms of depression, and that couples fare better than those who are on their own. We
know that taking the time to share our feelings with others can help us
to move through a difficult period. Sometimes, however, it is really hard
to take that step regardless of how close we might feel to our loved ones.
In case you have felt that reluctance, here is a story for you.

When my daughter, Melissa, was terribly ill and her future was
unknown, there was a time when I should have followed my own
advice and connected more deeply with friends and family. Instead, I
didn't ask for their help. If I could turn back the clock, I would handle
things in a different way. Travel with me now to that difficult period,
just in case you face something similar.

*Bouncing along the winding country road, my dirt-streaked Jeep
passes views of lush green fields sloping to sparkling waters, sailboats in the*

distance, and homes scattered along the shore. Pockets of poverty still remain in this land of affluence and indulgence, reminding us of misfortune, and how important it is to do all that we can to help the world.

My body and mind absorb the views of Blue Hill Bay, playing with thoughts of summers past, and just how things have changed. There is a destination/arrival desperation in me that stimulates my right foot to weigh heavily on the accelerator. Today I feel a sense of urgency to get to my husband to unload the last few days' woes. Today, "craves" is a word I would use to depict the need for comfort that I feel. It has been overwhelming. Weeks of visits to Dana Farber Cancer Institute with Melissa, sprinkled with thoughts that loom out of sleep and create 2 a.m. terror, have culminated in the creation of this deep, sorrowful, internal pit that desperately needs nurturing.

As I turn into our driveway, my face transitions from sadness to cheerily greet whatever family members might be gathered on the terrace on this perfect summer day. Ben and our daughter Kristin sit chatting, basking in the late summer sun that sparkles off the harbor, bordered by dozens of bobbing pink dahlias.

"How's Melissa doing?" Ben asks. Kristin, who tragically lost her mother at age four and knows about sadness, looks on hopefully. I can't break the spell of their day by being honest and I am not ready to dump my woes just yet. The vision of the most recent series of tubes and chemicals pumping into Melissa's body is just too fresh. And, I feel an unfamiliar resentment creeping in at how perfect this scene on the terrace was until I arrived. How unmarred by all that is happening to Melissa. This is unfair. Of course, they are deeply concerned and troubled by Melissa's cancer and all that she is enduring. But, sometimes all the trauma seems so outside of the rest of life—so far from this summer perfection at this wonderful cottage on the coast of Maine.

"Oh, okay I guess. She still isn't having any serious side effects from the chemo." I launch into an account of the trip to Dana Farber, leaving out the hours of sleepless nights, the overwhelming sense of sadness, and the tears.

"We were about to go kayaking," Ben says, "Are you going for a run?"

I look down at my spandex and running shoes and respond, "I guess." There are only two kayaks and it is a beautiful afternoon. They deserve to enjoy it. Ben and Kristin climb out of their chairs and head down the hill toward the dock. I wander around the cottage aimlessly for a while, not

*knowing what I want to do. I feel detached from everything, unable to plug
into the rest of my life, desperate to be cradled and comforted, not alone. I
scrawl a hasty note, put my bags back into the Jeep and leave.*

*The tears start to flow before I am barely a mile from the cottage, first
dripping, then pouring down my face, blurring my vision. "You have got
to get a grip on yourself," I say out loud as I continue on down the road.
"You are no good to anyone like this." For a couple of hours, I just drive.
Then I park and sit hopelessly looking out the window at the views of field
and ocean.*

*As I drive away, the tears come faster again, and I begin to howl. It is
a loud animal howl of pain that comes from so deep inside me that it feels
like it comes from another creature. I am gripping the steering wheel and
shaking so much that I need to pull over on the shoulder in order not to be
a highway hazard. I sit, sobbing and howling, feeling such huge sadness.
Still shaking, I pick up the cell phone and call my friend, Julie Merck. We
talk for a while about Melissa and about Julie's mother, whom she lost
shortly before I met her. She asks me to come to her house, but I am limp,
exhausted, a mess, and can't face any more driving. I thank her, we plan
a hike for the next morning, and I head the car toward Acadia National
Park. For now I am purged, thanks to the support of one of my many dear
friends. When I get home, I call Ben and tell him I'll be back at the cottage the next afternoon, knowing that by then I will be able to forge ahead
again. Sometimes, even when there are so many good people around, it feels
so lonely.*

So, there you have it. Within easy reach of people who loved me, I
pulled away. I just kept driving that Jeep on down the road. Please reach
out to the people you care about when you are feeling down. They will
welcome your request. When you ask for their assistance, you are essentially giving them encouragement to do the same thing with you when
they are in trouble. This is what reciprocal relationships are all about.

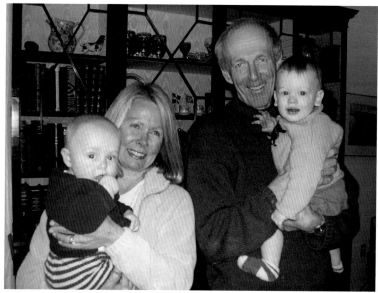

Sarah Wickenden

Spend Time with Those You Love.

EVALUATING YOUR SUPPORT SYSTEM

Throughout this book, I hope you will hear this message: In the same way that you are in the decision-making seat each day of your life, you are the most important part of your own treatment team when you are facing a challenging period. Through including your family members, friends, pets, medical professionals, and others in your support system, you can create a very powerful team that can mobilize many resources to help you to combat the presenting challenge, experience any treatments in a positive manner, and bring you to a healthier place.

If you were faced with a crisis or needed to bounce an idea off someone right now, who would it be? How about making a list of several people with whom you would feel comfortable sharing your feelings? In the best of situations, family and friends are critical to human health, but as we age and when we face challenges, they are even more important. It can be interesting to consider whether those whom you would call to share a hike or a movie are the same folks you would call on when you are scared or lonely.

Let's begin by thinking about the people that make up our support system and the elements in our lives that represent positive engagements. We can do this together, including all of the people and other entities that are important to us. In addition to family and friends, I am going to add Acadia National Park, Virgin Islands National Park, other green spaces, the ocean, my bike, my spiritual support system, my thinking mind, my running and hiking legs, my paddle boards, our home, my volunteer efforts at Maine Coast Heritage Trust and Schoodic Institute, my skis, the birds and other creatures, my memories, my imagination, my creativity, our cat, our access to the water in many ways, my gardens, my indoor green space and plants. You get the idea. Go for it.

All of the support system that we generate is available at every turn as we grow, and change, and age. Some elements come and go in their level of importance and some people drift in and out of our lives. We lose some from this world, but connect with them spiritually, and they help us in other ways. This entire system is miraculous, and holds great promise for us in all of our life encounters.

Now let's look at how we react when faced with a medical crisis. Building a support team can be a very important part of strengthening one's role in the treatment process. Most of us have experienced the anxiety related to waiting for test results. We are suspended in limbo until the reports come in. It is a dreadful time, when a sense of things being out of our control is at its highest. We pray, beg, and plead for everything to be fine. We agonize over all the possibilities, envisioning the prospects for what lies ahead, given different scenarios. We promise that, if our loved one's or our own diagnosis is a good one, we will lead cleaner lives, be nicer to the world and everyone in it, appreciate everyday…whatever it takes, just as long as we hear the "no" rather than the "yes."

And then, when the call comes, life hangs by a thread while the physician delivers the results. The power that my doctors held felt so familiar throughout my twenties when I had a series of biopsies for breast lumps. The anxiety has reappeared over the years many times as I have sat waiting. Have you felt this way, too? It seems that the receipt of final results always involves a weekend, so that the agony is extended.

In a few seconds, what is reported on that call can mean that life can return to normal or that it is thrown into a state of complete turmoil.

Our physicians and their medical support personnel are obviously critical to our treatment. It is not necessary, however, to turn over complete control to them or to make them larger than life. They are an important part of a team that we can create in order to empower ourselves throughout the treatment process. We want that team to be so forceful that it creates a strong and effective combat squad that can, hopefully, wipe out the ailment and restore us to full health.

If we include all of the medical specialists who are involved during the treatment of any case of cancer, the numbers are large. When I reflect on the first day that my daughter, Melissa, visited Dana Farber, I can count at least thirty people who directly participated in her case. Every one of them treated her like they had known her for years. Over the three years of her treatment and another ten of complications and follow-up, there were dozens more. If we consider each of those individuals a part of her treatment team, that is a very significant start in building a support system. Building upon the medical staff, if we include all of the treatments that modern medicine and mind/body approaches offered Melissa, another dimension of the team materializes. We can't forget all of those people who may not be in her inner circle, but who regularly express their caring and support.

Then, of course, there are those from Melissa's innermost circle: the friends and family members who are closest to her. Now, let's add Melissa's positive engagements at the time of her medical crisis and all of the activities that are important to her.

This is such a powerful, supportive, and nurturing team that it offers great strength in assisting with any present or future crisis. Go ahead. Build your team.

You might want to think first about your own support network of family, friends, and others. Start by making a list of all of those people as quickly as you can, then slow down and add those who were left out. Then make a list of your positive engagements. Now draw a circle and put your very closest companions, loved ones, and positive engagements in it. Then draw an outer circle and put the next tier of friends, family, and engagements within that. Then go one or two more circles out, placing more names of people and engagements you can count on. You can expand out as far as you choose.

KEEPING YOUR SPIRITUALITY TURNED ON

We all have deeply personal ways of expressing our spirituality. Whatever works for you, in whatever religion or manner of spiritual expression it manifests itself, is the route to follow. Personal healing and life direction can be so significantly impacted by the quality of our engagement with a higher power. More than ten years ago, research demonstrated that cardiac patients were less likely to die when specified caring individuals prayed for them, despite the fact that the patients were unaware of the experiment. Science also tells us that those who consider themselves to be religious live longer than those who don't and that praying lowers blood pressure. The relaxed state induced by prayer resembles other meditative states that have been documented as lowering blood pressure, reducing pain, and alleviating insomnia.

It feels important to share with you the fact that I pray repeatedly throughout the day and night. There is a thankfulness prayer that spills forth frequently whether I am running, waking in the night, paddle boarding, gardening, driving, or doing one of a thousand other things. It relates to thankfulness for each element in our natural world, thankfulness for my family and friends, and thankfulness for the time I have been given to work on behalf of our world and her creatures. It includes a pledge to do the best that I can to help to care for all. If it feels like someone else needs some assistance, I ask for help for that person or help for the world itself. Is there a way that you do something similar? My approach follows.

Thank you for this second, this minute, this hour, this day, this week, this month, this year, this life. Thank you for giving me more than I ever expected.

Thank you for the sky, the universe, the planets, the sun, the moon, the stars, the earth, the clouds, and thank you for the air that we breathe. Thank you for the sunshine, the rain, the snow, the sleet, the hail, and the breezes.

Thank you for the creatures of the sky—the birds, the bees, the butter-flies, the moths, the bats, the insects, and all the other creatures of the sky. I will do the best that I can to help to care for your world and your creatures.

Thank you for the earth and for the soil. Thank you for the geological features. Thank you for the things that grow on the earth and in the soil. Thank you for the fruits, the berries, the vegetables, the trees and the shrubs, the flowers and the plants, the weeds and the grasses, the lichens and the mosses, and all the other things that grow on your earth and in your soil. I will do the best I can to help to care for your world and your creatures.

Thank you for the creatures of the earth and of the soil. Thank you for the reptiles, the amphibians, the mammals, the birds, the worms, the crustaceans, the insects, and all the other creatures of your earth and of your soil. I will do the best that I can to help to care for your world and your creatures.

Thank you for the waters, fresh and salt. Thank you for the lakes and the ponds, the rivers and the streams, the bogs and the brooks, the marshes and the swamps, the estuaries and the salt ponds, and thank you for the oceans wide that bind us all together.

Thank you for the creatures of your waters, fresh and salt. Thank you for the fishes, the birds, the mammals, the reptiles, the amphibians, the worms, the crustaceans, the insects, and all the other creatures of your waters, fresh and salt. I will do the best that I can to help to care for your world and your creatures.

Thank you for my family and for my friends. Thank you for strengthening them and caring for them physically, emotionally, and spiritually, helping them to do the best that they can do to help to care for your world and your creatures. I will do the best that I can to help to care for each of them. (Here I list individuals, mentioning specifics about them.)

Thank you for giving me much more time than I ever expected to work on behalf of your world and your creatures. Thank you for guiding me spiritually, emotionally, and physically. Thank you for helping me to hear your wisdom, your guidance, your direction, and your encouragement. Thank you for guiding my thoughts, my words, my thinking, my writing, my speaking, my purpose, my creativity, my direction, my goals, and my actions. I will do the best that I can to help to care for your world and your creatures.

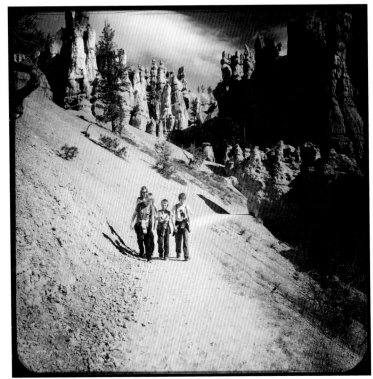

Jamie Schapiro

Bathed in Ethereal Light: Bryce Canyon National Park.

JOURNALING

Did you know that those who write about distressing events have stronger immune systems and visit their doctors about half as much as those who write only about trivial events? In the mid-90's, researchers at Southern Methodist University found that journaling has these physical benefits as well as the more frequently documented emotional benefits of relieving stress and depression. Earlier, we focused on writing about concerns as one antidote for sleep difficulties that swirl around worries. The more you write to express your feelings, the easier it will become, and the more impact it will have. In the process of repetitive writing, our writing becomes better, too.

Putting your thoughts on paper does help to release them. It also helps you to build upon them. Computers are especially effective, as you can so easily move things around and delete items that don't feel like a fit. Putting something in writing does not mean that you are wedded to it or need to keep it. Generating written material is sometimes difficult because, like any form of art, writing is a statement about oneself, and it can be very hard to take the step of opening that self up to criticism. Let's think about that in a different way. We don't need to share our writing with others if we don't choose to. When we open ourselves up and do release our writing to others, it is very similar to sharing ourselves in other ways. In making that intimate gesture, we are also giving others permission to take a risk with us, thus granting one another an opportunity to bond in the relationship. Your writing can lead you in this direction. Or, you can use it for self-expression and venting and then just keep it for yourself. I am really glad I kept my childhood and teen diaries as they have given me great insight into the person that I was during difficult times. They have also allowed me to share stories that I hope you will find helpful. What do you think about trying a little writing right now? If you need a topic, you might write about a time when someone shared a personal experience with you.

THE LAUGHTER AND HAPPINESS PRESCRIPTION

"Laughter is a form of internal jogging." Lee Berk, DrPH,
Professor of Pathology and Anatomy, Linda Loma University

Jogging along the Eagle Lake carriage road on a warm spring day, I step into an apparent branch that trips me up. Turning to move it, I discover a large troupe of panicked two-foot snakes scattering in every direction. Clearly, my feet have landed in a ball of copulating, but thankfully non-poisonous, snakes. There is no shortage of laughter as my run continues and I then repeat the tale numerous times, including that evening at a dinner party where one guest nearly loses his dinner.

Running on the streets of South Florida can get one outside safely, as long as you pay attention. My mind drifts away as I become caught up in thoughts and mentally transport myself to another place.

Racing along, I suddenly register that there is something going on up ahead on the sidewalk. An army of orange-helmeted workmen, draped over pick-axes and shovels, greets me enthusiastically with cat calls and whistles. Smugly, I note that I am probably older than their mothers and vainly revel in this thought. Noticing their three-foot wide trench just in time, I leap over it, hearing their Latino chorus as I hit mid-air. Landing on the other side of the marked work area, my feet hit mush, and I am sucked rapidly downward into thick, slimy mud. Before I can react, those South Florida Spanish voices are around me, the brawny arms of their owners grabbing at me and scooping me out of the muck. A high pressure hose hits me full force, the hands of many men scrub my body, and I detect the word, "cement" as my rescuers attempt to clean me off. I have plunged feet-first into a manhole that has been filled with fresh cement.

Thanking my new-found friends, and laughing somewhat hysterically at the level of intimacy that we have established, I slog back to my daughter, Bethany's. Sopping wet from the top of my head down to the sidewalk, I ring her bell and present myself in my cement shoes. "Now what have you done?" she asks.

Three gray squirrels scurry up our screen door, skitter their way across the thin wire that supports our bird feeders, then take turns extricating seeds while hanging by one foot and a tail. They have foiled us again, and we laugh at their success.

Some rattling wakes me at 1 AM, encouraging me to peek out through the drapes to watch a large raccoon, balanced carefully on his robust friend, as he turns the seed tube attached to our feeder wire upside down, and pours birdseed into his mouth.

Two chasing chipmunks, intent on romance, run up the leg of a shocked picnic guest, across his chest, and down the other side.

Direct encounters with nature can bring us much laughter, as can videos of kids and animals, a good joke, cartoons, and so many other experiences. Numerous studies show that smiling promotes the release of mood-enhancing endorphins within our brains. As French novelist and playwright Victor Hugo once said, "Laughter is the sun that drives winter from the human face." Back in the early 2000s there was an explosion of research related to happiness, optimism, and laughter. At this point in time, that seems to be happening again. We can always use a good laugh. As I write this, I glance at my screen to discover that spell-check has corrected the word "happiness" in my writing to "hairiness." That was enough to stimulate a laugh. Did you just hear my laughter as it lowered the release of cortisol, the primary stress hormone? Have you been laughing or smiling in the last few minutes, too?

How about making a list of some times when you have had a good laugh? What about laughter's close ally, happiness? Are you happy a good bit of the time? Would you like to find some ways to bring more happiness into your life?

Research by the deans of happiness research, Martin Seligman, Ph.D., and Edward Deiner, Ph.D., found that the most prominent characteristic shared by those with the lowest levels of depression and the highest levels of happiness were their "strong ties to friends and family and commitment to spending time with them."[7]

The Satisfaction with Life Scale
To evaluate levels of happiness, Deiner, Emmons, Larsen, and Griffin developed a five question survey that is now internationally employed, *The Satisfaction with Life Scale*.[8]

Use a seven (strongly agree) to a one (strongly disagree) rating:
    7—strongly agree
    6—agree
    5—slightly agree
    4—neither agree nor disagree
    3—slightly disagree
    2—disagree
    1—strongly disagree

Use the 7 to 1 rating of your level of agreement with these five questions:
    _____ In most ways my life is close to my ideal.
    _____ The conditions of my life are excellent.
    _____ I am satisfied with my life.
    _____ So far I have gotten the important things I want in life.
    _____ If I could live my life over, I would change almost nothing.

Compute a total score.
    31-35: You are extremely satisfied with your life.
    26-30: Very satisfied.
    21-25: Slightly satisfied.
    20 is the neutral point.
    15-19: Slightly dissatisfied.
    10-14: Dissatisfied.
    5-9: Extremely dissatisfied.

Seligman found that of three components of happiness, 1) pleasure (pursuit of pleasure); 2) engagement (the depth of engagement with one's work, family, hobbies, and romance); and 3) meaning (using personal strength to serve some larger end), engagement and meaning are much more consequential than pleasure. Seligman, researcher Sonja Lyubomirsky, Ph.D.[89], and psychologist Dr. Robert Emmons[90] also learned in separate studies that the most effective ways to boost happiness are to express gratitude to others; to perform acts of kindness; to be aware of your blessings by writing down three positive experiences each day; to identify your strengths and find ways to use them; to practice forgiveness; to spend time with friends and family; to care for your body; to learn approaches to dealing with stress and hardships.

This good advice can be taken a step further if we establish a self-fulfilling prophecy each morning: This day will hold goodness. I will be grateful for even small good things. And, I will do at least one good thing for someone else.

For the times when we need an extra boost, let's assemble a list of resources of scenes and stories that will give us positive feelings or a good laugh, or let's go online to watch some funny videos. We might find ourselves in circumstances where they won't take away unpleasantness forever, but they can give us a break and a release of tension. Research has demonstrated that those who enjoy humor report being less lonely, less stressed, and less anxious than those who don't joke. A happy attitude, or optimism, was found to correlate with longevity.[9]

Credit for boosting happiness has been given to the world and its creatures for quite some time. A report generated by Frederick Law Olmsted in 1865 related to the status of Yosemite stated that reinvigoration from nature "not only gives pleasure for the time being but increases the subsequent capacity for happiness and the means of securing happiness." We also know that 1) positive feelings correlate with levels of exercise on a daily basis, particularly in the green outdoors; 2) that our feelings can be affected by what we put into our bodies; 3) that we do better when we have positive relationships; 4) that relaxation and visualization can impact levels of positive feelings; 5) that volunteer experiences lead to a greater degree of life satisfaction; and that 6) "a core set of beliefs that are not easily shattered"[10] can help us to be more resilient. The recipe for happiness and laughter is consistent with that for the other goals we are addressing.

Fast forwarding to 2017, we find some sound scientific research spearheaded by Dr. Judith Moskowitz[11], who assembled a set of eight approaches that help to promote positive emotions. Pilot studies indicated that caregivers of dementia patients as well as women with advanced stage breast cancer demonstrated a decrease in depression after participation in the positive emotions training course. "Having a positive view of aging can have a beneficial influence on health outcomes and longevity,"[11] according to a study of 4,000 people age 50+ at the Yale School of Public Health, published in 2016 in the *Journal of Gerontology*. Researcher Dr. Becca Levy also stated, "Psychologically, a positive view can enhance belief in one's abilities, decrease perceived stress, and foster healthful behaviors. Physiologically, people with positive views of aging had lower levels of C-reactive protein, a marker of stress-related inflammation associated with heart disease and other illnesses, even after accounting for possible influences like age, health status, sex, race, and education than those with a negative outlook. They also lived significantly longer."[12] Personally, I take these words as very encouraging. I am far from an expert in many of the subjects in which I engage, but I have two great secrets. First is the fact that my relationships include many remarkable individuals who are experts in multitudinous fields. They, who have taught me so much, are a resource to which I turn when I am seeking wisdom. There is one spot, however, where I am quite confident that I am in the top 1%. That is in aging happily and in my boundless appreciation for life and the world around me—the root of our shared journey. Thank you, God and the Universe, for giving me this second secret as well as so many experiences—the uplifting as well as the challenging—and for helping me to pass the benefit of my journey on to others.

NUTRITION: EATING OUR WAY
TO GOOD HEALTH

"Come forth into the light of things, let nature be your teacher."
William Wordsworth

You are going to love this little nugget from my memory. Somewhere along the line, I read a study of rats and nutrition. My apologies go through the ethers to the scientists who conducted this study, as I can nowhere find reference to it now. As we think about good nutrition and the impact that it has on how we feel and how we act, this rat study is a great illustration of the dire consequences that dietary choices can have for our behavior. We do know that we are a lot like rats, and that some of us may be more rat-like than others. For three months, four groups of rats were fed four different diets. The rats that were fed natural foods and clean water (group 1) remained alert, curious, and calm. The rat group that dined only on hotdogs and water (group 2) became violent, fighting aggressively and biting off their own tails. Some even bit off their own tongues. The rats that ate sugar doughnuts and drank cola (group 3) slept fitfully. They did not huddle with their rat friends, as rats normally would do, but instead hunkered quivering in corners, unable to function as a social unit. When approached from outside the cage, they became extremely fearful. The rats that ate sugar-coated cereal and drank fruit punch (group 4) ran around and around their cage in a hyperactive, aimless, and nervous manner. Some hung upside down from their little rat homes. Hmm. We could take some lessons from that study, whether we are old folks, young folks, sick folks, or busy folks.

Alarmingly, a 2016 study, published in Mayo Clinic Proceedings and based on data gathered from the National Health and Nutrition Survey that included a nationally representative sample of 4,745 Americans, found that "fewer than 3% of American adults follow the heart-healthy lifestyle of eating a healthful diet (eating plenty of fruits and vegetables and whole grains and avoiding saturated fat), not smoking, being physically active (at least 150 minutes of moderate exercise a week), and keeping weight and body fat (20% for men and 30% for women) down."[13]

We all slip up and inhale the six cookies or bag of Goldfish occasionally. We don't need to beat ourselves up about it, but it would behoove us to pay attention to some of the information that we see time and time again. It will make a difference because we are, indeed, what we eat. A helpful note from McGill University suggests breaking food cravings by looking out a window at the natural world or by interacting with an animal. So, focus on a nearby tree or garden and pat your puppy.

Aren't we fortunate that our green outdoors and our indoor green spaces can provide some of the vegetables, nuts, and fruits that contribute to our good health? When we are engaging with plants in our environment, which provides many physical and emotional benefits, we can also access the foods that will strengthen our bodies and our minds. Foraging in the wild and growing a bounty of foods in one's own garden are satisfying endeavors. Wouldn't it be great to grow our own fruits and vegetables inside our homes as well? Oh, you lucky people with greenhouses or warm climates! Then, I think of our friends, Eliot Coleman and Barbara Damrosch. Eliot broke all the assumptions to bits and developed an internationally-renowned year-round organic farm in downeast Maine with five acres of land and a mini hoop house system that he designed himself. Barbara joined Eliot many years ago, producing a brilliant and hard-working team who do not mind getting their hands dirty. Prolific authors and teachers, Eliot and Barbara's books are beautifully written guides to producing and presenting the Earth's bounty. They are generous with their time, willingly sharing it with audiences and nonprofits, as well as the interns they mentor. And, they brought us the best carrots I have ever eaten straight out of the soil—in November!

In this era of health awareness, we are constantly bombarded with information about what we should and should not be eating to avoid illness and to reduce our level of stress. While common sense could probably go a long way in helping to protect us, there is some basic advice available that we should all heed. First, let's take a lesson from the birds who pursue food as fuel. If we were able to do that, the perpetual obesity epidemic in our country would likely be a non-issue. We would also avoid many of the ailments that are related to obesity and the resulting costs to society. But, let's take where we are right now and try to work toward a healthier place.[94, 95, 96, 97, 98, 99]

We know that low-fat diets filled with vegetables, fruits, and fiber encourage a healthy body and mind and that there are also foods that we would do well to avoid. Nurturing the body through a healthy diet can help to keep us physically robust and on an even emotional keel. When we are experiencing stressful life periods, choosing the right foods can make the difference between coping adequately and falling apart. This does not mean abandoning all of the foods we enjoy and subsequently feeling deprived. Instead, it means developing an awareness of which foods can most significantly impact our emotions, making educated choices about what we put into our bodies, and making some adjustments during stressful periods.

As we are aging or during a medical crisis, we can gain an active and powerful role in the process through giving ourselves proper nutrition and paying attention to foods that can nurture our emotions. When I am going through a difficult period, one food that I include in my diet regularly is spinach, a vegetable that has a direct link to alleviating depression. Vitamin B-rich foods are believed to synthesize brain chemicals, very low levels of which may induce depression. Asparagus, winter squash, pinto beans, baked potatoes, salmon, bananas, tuna, cheese, and meat are all part of a healthy mood-elevating diet.

The production of serotonin, which has been linked to the alleviation of depression, can be stimulated through the consumption of complex carbohydrates. Grains, root vegetables, pasta, and fruits all fall into this category. When these foods are not combined with high-fat foods and/or protein, they induce drowsiness and assist in relaxation, so if it's sleepiness you are looking for, dine on carbs. Beans, nuts, and seeds added to your diet will supply the copper and iron that are also important for good sleep. Half an ounce of low-fat cheese or some mixed nuts before bedtime contain the amino acid tryptophan, a component of serotonin, which induces sleep. Tension-reducing foods include wheat germ, carrots, broccoli, red bell peppers, oranges, strawberries, and apricots. If you have trouble with restless leg syndrome, pumpkin seeds and leafy greens contain magnesium, which can relax your muscles. A deficiency in calcium, which can result in numbness in fingers and toes, as well as muscle cramping, can be avoided through consumption of sardines, milk, yogurt, cheese, and dark green leafy vegetables.

Foods that can help to alleviate fatigue due to their potassium and phosphorus content include cottage cheese, bananas, and carrots. If you are hoping to replace some of your meat consumption with vegetables, those highest in energy-boosting protein include lima beans, sprouted lentils, peas, beans, and kale.

If each day we were to consume even a fraction of the foods I have just mentioned, it is hard to believe that we would have any room left for those products that can cause us problems. Old habits die hard, however, and many of us were well-indoctrinated into the "feed your feelings syndrome" during our youth. Offered as rewards for good behavior, expressions of affection, and something to look forward to, cookies, candies, cakes, and their sweet cousins beckon us to indulge. Although we do not need to walk away from these goodies completely, for many reasons their consumption should be limited. The brief highs followed by discouraging lows that they produce will not help us when we are trying to keep our energy up and our emotions in balance. Is it really worth consuming fried foods, sugar, refined cereals, and processed meat when dozens of research studies demonstrate that their consumption correlates with depressed feelings?

The first two adjustments I make to my diet when I am going through a tough period are to give up sugar and alcohol. I know well that, for me, both of these products result in sleep disruption, decreased energy, and a low mood. Even my one little glass of wine before dinner can send me off to a sound sleep, only to wake long before dawn with what I call "two o'clock terror." For some reason, everything seems worse in the middle of the night. I like getting up at 4:00, but I do not like ending a night's sleep at 2 AM.

According to numerous physicians who have written about the food-mood connection, chronic hypoglycemia—or low blood sugar—creates symptoms that include depression, anxiety, fatigue, irritability, mood swings, and difficulty in concentrating. Foods to avoid include simple carbohydrates like refined sugar, honey, white flour, and canned fruit in syrup, as well as alcohol, caffeine, and artificial sweeteners.

Dieticians and physicians suggest small meals and frequent healthy snacks that include nuts, fish, fowl, and meats that supply protein; complex carbohydrates like whole grains and legumes, fresh vegetables, and fresh fruits; and a modest amount of low-fat dairy that includes plain yogurt. Numerous studies report that fewer symptoms of depression were indicated in those who consumed primarily fish, fruits, vegetables, and whole grains.[92]

Fluid retention related to overuse of salt causes sluggishness and irritability for many people. Furthermore, there is a risk of developing hypertension if sodium is consumed in large quantities. Just what is a "large quantity" of salt? The Food and Nutrition Board of the National Academy of Sciences has established the minimum amount of sodium per day for healthy adults at 500 mg and the maximum amount at 2,300 mg. One teaspoon of salt contains about 2,300 mg of sodium. In their natural state, most foods contain some sodium. It is likely that we reach our minimum advised daily level without adding salt to anything. Many processed foods represent sodium out of control, particularly lunch meats, fast foods, frozen dinners, and canned goods to which salt has been added. *Elsevier* reports in its journal, *Appetite*, that people leaving fast food restaurants who were asked to guess how much sodium they had just consumed guessed 200 mg, on the average. The actual average was 1,300 mg. Healthy substitutes for table salt include pepper, garlic, lemon, herbs, or spices.

When we are fatigued, it is important to determine if we are dehydrated. Clear-colored, yellow-tinged urine indicates good hydration; dark urine indicates dehydration. Other signs of dehydration include extreme thirst, confusion, fatigue, dizziness, and less frequent urination. Regular consumption of water is critical to good health and energy levels. Electrolytes, the salts your body needs for proper functioning, are often lost during exercise, illness, and travel. The electrolytes sodium, chloride, and potassium are essential to maintaining proper hydration. An imbalance and the related dehydration can result in muscle cramping, fatigue, numbness, and irregular heartbeat. Foods high in electrolytes include soymilk, seafood, cheese, and yogurt. Those containing potassium, such as dark green leafy vegetables, potatoes, beans, bananas, yogurt, fish, and squash and those containing magnesium like fish, Swiss chard, kale, spinach, seeds, and nuts all help to balance electrolytes. When exercising heavily, particularly in hot climates, we sip a bit of Gatorade every now and then, along with plenty of water. According to Gatorade, the drink encourages water consumption and its sodium "helps maintain body fluids without promoting water loss through increased urination."

Over the years, too many times new patients appeared in my office with a diagnosis of unsuccessfully-treated anxiety disorder that actually related to caffeine overdose. Some of these individuals moved on and off a number of medications, spent thousands of dollars on therapy, suffered for years, and, in a few cases, were hospitalized in psychiatric institutions. Their symptoms included irritability, restlessness, sleep disruption, heart palpitations, trembling, panic, and gastrointestinal difficulties. When questioned about her diet, one extremely distressed woman reported drinking forty cups of coffee a day. In all her years of difficulties, no one had ever asked about her caffeine intake. For some individuals any amount of caffeine can cause anxiety, insomnia, trembling, and/or irritability. The average adult can consume two six-ounce cups of brewed coffee (200 mg) before exhibiting some degree of caffeine toxicity. One rounded teaspoon of instant coffee contains 57 mg of caffeine, one rounded teaspoon of decaffeinated coffee contains 2 mg, six fluid ounces of tea which is steeped for three minutes has 36 mg, 12 fluid ounces of diet or regular Coke contains 46 mg, and one ounce of chocolate contains 12 mg. Bear in mind as well that 2017 research indicates that consumption of even one diet soda a day may increase the risk of stroke and dementia due to the sweetener, not the caffeine. When we are coping with stressful life events or exhibiting any of the symptoms described above, it is especially important to assess our caffeine intake. Lowering our consumption might help us to handle our lives more comfortably.

Mood Foods

For the fun and education of it, here is a collection of foods that may have positive ramifications for your body and your mind. Unless we are allergic, they will surely do no harm as we age or undergo stress. Please consult your physician if you are experiencing difficulties with anxiety, pain, fatigue, stress, depression, or illness. While dietary changes can be helpful, they may be only a part of the puzzle.[94, 95, 96, 97, 98, 99]

Foods to Help with Relaxation
potatoes, root vegetables, popcorn, pasta,
rices, whole grains, cereal (any high fats/protein eaten within
4 hours of carbs will negate their sleepiness effect), seeds, nuts
(high fructose corn syrup on nuts interferes with copper absorption),
tofu, dried fruit, beans, peas, spinach, dark greens,
shellfish, red meat (Vitamin C increases iron absorption)

Foods to Help with Pain Relief
seeds, nuts (high fructose corn syrup on nuts interferes with copper absorption), spinach, sardines, salmon, almonds, skim milk, yogurt, cheese, nuts, seeds, whole grain pasta, whole grain bread

Foods to Help Alleviate Fatigue
sardines, salmon, chicken, beef, beans, nuts, tofu

Foods to Help Combat Stress
bananas, dried fruits, oranges, strawberries, apples,
carrots, spinach, red bell peppers, beans

Foods to Help Fight Depression
salmon, sardines, tuna, other oily fish, walnuts, flaxseed, leafy greens, seafood, spinach, asparagus, beans, seeds, parsley,
winter squash, wheat germ, chicken, meat (in small amounts)

Foods to Help Protect the Body from Illness
eggs, meat, lima beans, oysters, clams, wheat germ, safflower and

sunflower oils, spinach, leafy green vegetables, lentils, beans, peas, broccoli, cabbage, dried fruits, bananas, avocados, chicken, carrots, citrus fruits, brussel sprouts, strawberries, sardines, other fatty fish, sweet potatoes, figs, cantaloupe

Looking for a way to lose weight and stay healthy? Try this.
Before eating anything else in a day, feed yourself from this list.
(Throughout the day, drink your RDA of water):
1 cup of cooked oatmeal with ½ a chopped apple, ¼ cup frozen blueberries, and some low-sugar cranberries mixed in while cooking. More fresh fruit and soymilk or skim milk added before serving.
1 cup of berries
1 cup lowfat plain or fruit yogurt
1 cup of cooked leafy greens (spinach, kale, beet greens, chard, etc.)
½ cup of cooked beans, lima beans, peas, or asparagus
½ cup of squash
½ cup of carrots
1 tomato
1 can of sardines
1 orange
1 banana
another fruit of your choice
another vegetable of your choice
1 serving salmon, trout, chicken, eggs, sprouted lentils, peas, or beans
⅛ cup sunflower seeds

Hints to Make Foods Healthier:
Use soymilk in soups and sauces.
Use skim or low fat milk.
Use two egg whites instead of one egg in recipes.
Use yogurt in place of mayonnaise.
Avoid refined sugar and flour.
Purchase low sodium foods and canned goods.
Avoid imitation meats.
Avoid prepared foods so that you know what is going into your body.

My favorite hiking, biking, or trail run energy foods are sardines packed in spring water, nuts, Nature Valley granola bars, and yogurt in a Ziploc bag. Bite off a little corner of the baggie (save it to put in the trash later), and squeeze the yogurt into your mouth. Be sure the baggie is zipped tight first! For running or hiking, carrying a bottle of water in each hand works very well. This is in addition to what is in the backpack. You can start with the little bottles, move on to the 700 ml variety, and then to the five liter size. This really keeps the old arm muscles up to speed. We do not use my weight bottles for drinking unless we run out of everything else. In the tropics or the desert, don't forget the Gatorade.

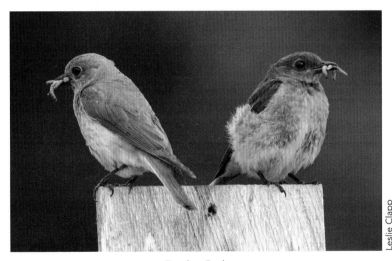

Food as Fuel.

Leslie Clapp

EXERCISE: THE BEST OF IT
IN THE GREEN OUTDOORS

"In every walk with nature one receives more than he seeks."
John Muir

Laughter explodes from the group of young ones as they race up Dorr Mountain's granite steps for the twentieth time in ten weeks. This therapy group for children, whose parents are recovering substance abusers, gathers at our local hospital. Twice a week, I take them to Acadia National Park for some outdoor exercise that will help them physically and emotionally. Therapy in the Park works well for all ages, producing the added benefits of physical fitness, increased self-esteem, and contact with nature. It is 1988 when we start this particular group, a time when therapy in nature doesn't often take place. Here on Mount Desert Island, home of Acadia National Park, it is a natural.

Mount Desert Island Hospital, where I served on the Allied Health Professional Staff, asked that I design and implement a counseling program for young children of substance abusers who were attending the hospital's outpatient substance abuse treatment program. In order to most effectively and efficiently meet the needs of these children, I set up a program that would incorporate group therapy, coping skills, substance abuse education, healthy lifestyle education, active outdoor engagement, social interaction and bonding with peers, and controlled risk activities (hiking a mountain) for self-concept development.

This group of 8 to 12 year-olds moaned and groaned their way up Dorr Mountain for the first three weeks. Frequent calls included, "I can't do it!" "I hate this!" "My legs hurt." Several weeks down the road, all were trotting merrily up the steps, examining plants and trees along the way, and delighting in occasional sightings of wildlife. Their self-esteem scores had sky-rocketed, their bodies hiked the hillside with ease, they had learned some things about the natural world and its creatures, they had formed important peer relationships, and they were coping better with the challenges of home and school. Success, thanks to exercise and green therapy in the natural world!

The feelings that are generated by thoughts of that group lead me to report on a quite extraordinary physical education teacher and coach. After a springtime of hiking his oft-complaining eighth graders around Acadia National Park, an especially hot day saw them climbing Sargent Mountain, moaning and groaning as much as those kids from the hospital group that I just told you about. As they neared Sargent Mountain Pond, exhausted and sweating, Coach Herb Watson laughed, "Bet you guys would love a cold Coke right now." More moans ensued as Herb leapt into the bushes and reappeared with a case of Coke that he had climbed the mountain to deliver before dawn. Do you think any of those kids, now in their fifties, ever forgot that? Do you think they were inspired to continue throughout life to get themselves and their loved ones out into the great outdoors?

According to the Centers for Disease Control and Prevention, fewer than 25% of American adults get the recommended amount of aerobic exercise and strength training each week. It is shocking to acknowledge that the average American child spends only four to seven minutes each day in unstructured outdoor play and more than seven hours a day in front of an electronic screen. The American Academy of Pediatrics recommends a minimum of 60 minutes of unstructured play per day. The significant benefits of outdoor exercise for children include stress levels that fall within minutes of seeing green spaces.[14] Dr. Robin Puett of the Maryland Institute for Applied Environmental Health conducted a large-scale study that concluded that people who exercised partially or entirely outdoors exercised more. Puett stated, "Our study suggests that exercising outdoors, whether alone or combined with indoor physical activity, may be linked to better self-perception of health and emotional outlook, as well as reduced tension, for women and more active adults."[15]

A growing body of medical research began to build in the early 2000s, and by 2005 the American Psychological Association was endorsing exercise as a legitimate third form of treatment for depression, along with psychotherapy and medication. Several studies demonstrated that, in addition to the renowned endorphin-releasing "runners' high" that produces a temporary lift, continued relief from a depressed mood can set in after several weeks in a regular exercise program. That is substantiating evidence for those of us who know in our hearts that aerobic activity, in particular, helps us to feel well and that any exercise in the outdoors is a terrific mood enhancer. In regard to those who are prescribed medication for depression, Harvard Medical School clinical professor of psychiatry, Dr. Douglas Jacobs, stated, "Between 20% and 30% of depression patients don't respond to medication after a year of taking it."[16] With symptoms of depression, a complete diagnostic evaluation and mood stabilization are essential, particularly given the fact that depression is the primary cause of suicide, one of the top several causes of death.

More recently, the February 2016 issue of *Neuroscience and Biobehavioral Reviews* reports on the analysis of twenty past studies in which blood samples were obtained from individuals with major depression before and after they exercised. Results indicated that "exercise significantly reduced various markers of inflammation and increased levels of a number of different hormones and other biochemicals that are thought to contribute to brain health."[17]

A study reported in *Preventive Medicine* of 1,140,000 adults was aimed at assessing whether exercise could act as a depression preventative. Several large-scale studies met the criteria with pre- and post-study objective measures of the participants' aerobic fitness and standardized evaluations of their mental health. Results indicated that men and women with the lowest level of fitness were 75% more likely to have been diagnosed with major depression than those who were most fit.[18] In addition, a study in the *Journal of Psychiatric Review* reported that moderately strenuous exercise, like jogging or brisk walking, had a significant effect on depression according to twenty-five pooled studies, with mental health improving considerably if participants diagnosed with depression were exercising.[19]

Any exercise in any environment will have benefits, but research is on the side of outdoor exercise in a green environment,[100, 101, 102, 103, 104, 105] as opposed to exercising indoors or on a city sidewalk with no trees. Green environments, defined by Kaplan in 1995 as "any environment that affords an individual the opportunity to view a more green type of scenery,"[20] have been shown to have greater impact on well-being, including increased energy, ability to concentrate, and ability to cope with stress. Decreased confusion, anger, depression, and tension were also reported.

What about the times when we cannot get outside? Then we position ourselves by a window with a view of green, amidst our indoor plants, in front of a lovely painting of the natural world, or we tune into a video with scenes of nature. We do whatever level of exercise feels appropriate for us. We know that people self-selecting the pace of their activities are more likely to enjoy and continue the engagements. Any level of activity and any degree of connection with the natural world and its creatures will help.

Sometimes, we all feel really desperate to get that burst of good, clean outdoor exercise. My friend, Cody VanHeerden, and I laugh as we recall the day that we set off on our cross-country skis only to find that conditions were so sticky that we had a foot of snow hanging off the length of our skis. Determined to get in our daily aerobic workout, we threw our skis in the bushes and ran six miles in our ski boots.

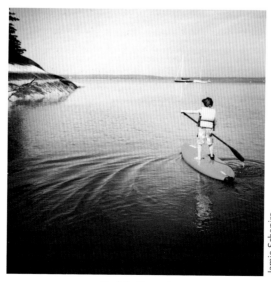

Jamie Schapiro

Paddle Power.

Stretches for Health and Fitness

When we consider pro-active approaches to health care, proper stretching is near the top of the list. It can help us relax, avoid injury, strengthen our backs, and return to a fit level. Most of us know what it is like to have a sore back, muscle strain, or post-surgery period. A downhill skiing injury sent me into recovery mode for eight weeks and set me up for several more exacerbations that were precipitated by events ranging from reaching for a garden plant to squatting for two hours while we cleaned our attic. Each time, these exercises helped me to strengthen with the help of a wonderful chiropractor and orthopedist. The greatest salvation came several years ago when I began stand-up paddle boarding. As it brings every part of your body into a fit state, one of the greatest benefits is to your back. It has now been five years since I have had a twinge.

Please resist the temptation to race through your exercises. Instead, make this some of your quiet time. You can even integrate some of your visualization and relaxation techniques while you are stretching. Keep your breathing slow and easy. Don't hold your breath or bounce up and down while stretching. Stretch only until you feel mild tension and relax as you hold the stretch for 10 to 30 seconds, silently counting the stretch time. These strengthening exercises are appropriate as a part of your lifetime fitness plan, as well as prior to and following surgery. Begin the exercises at the level that feels appropriate and that your doctor approves. Gradually increase them to repetitions of ten or more.

If you are recovering from surgery, check in with your physician and gradually begin your exercises again, keeping in mind that you should not push yourself too fast. Assist your body in the recovery process by performing four to eight repetitions of the first six exercises twice a day. Do not strain yourself or increase the number of repetitions more often than once a week. Add the other routines as you feel more comfortable, increasing repetitions of all exercises as you return to full health. Before beginning any exercise program, check with your physician and use his/her suggested number of repetitions.

Exercise 1

Feet 1' apart, arms parallel to the floor. Keeping arms in this position, reach toward the left side of the body with both arms. Toe in with the right foot to release knee pressure. Reverse.

Exercise 2
Feet 1' apart, arms at sides. With palms up, raise arms as high as possible. With palms down, slowly lower arms. Repeat.

Exercise 3
Feet 1' apart, hands together in front of body. Slowly, bring arms over the head in a circle. Palms up, lower arms to shoulder height. Turn palms down and lower to starting position. Repeat.

Exercise 4
Feet 1' apart, arms stretched out from sides at shoulder height. With left arm, reach as high as possible over head while looking at extended right arm. Return arms to starting position and reverse.

Exercise 5
Feet 1' apart, arms flexed at shoulder height. Keeping elbows at shoulder height, gently pull both elbows back, hold, then return to original position.

Exercise 6
Lying down with knees bent, lower back pressed to floor, feet flat on surface, arms at sides, palms up. Keeping fingers on surface throughout motion, bring arms as close to over head as possible. Slowly return to starting position.

Exercise 7
Lying flat on the floor, press back to floor while pulling right knee to chest and straightening left leg. Hold 5 seconds. Relax and repeat. Repeat with opposite leg.

Exercise 8
Lying on floor with knees bent, feet flat on floor, arms at sides, palms down, tighten lower abdomen and buttocks, flattening lower back. Slowly raise low back and buttocks. Hold 5 seconds, relax, and repeat.

Exercise 9
Lying on back with knees bent, feet flat on floor, hands at sides, palms down, tighten muscles of abdomen and buttocks, pushing low back flat against floor. Hold 5 seconds, relax, and repeat.

Exercises 1-6 were adapted by Eastern Maine Medical Center's Breast Center from a home exercise sheet prepared by Linda Morneault for the Bangor/Brewer, ME, YWCA ENCORE Program.

Exercises 7-9 are adapted from "Exercises to Rehabilitate and Strengthen the Low Back," prepared by Louis Sportelli, D.C., PO Box 213, Palmerton, PA 18071-0213.

Calories Burned (based on 130-pound woman)
Activity/Calories Burned per Hour

Running (9 minute mile) 684
Stand-up paddle boarding 600
Swimming a slow crawl 456
Hiking up hill 426
Cross-country skiing 420
Tennis 384
Weight training 330
Golf 300
Walking at a normal pace 282
Weeding the garden 252
Biking at 5.5 mph 228
Cleaning 222

5

VIEWING OTHERS' SUCCESSES

"Everybody needs beauty as well as bread,
places to play in and pray in, where nature may heal
and give strength to body and soul."
John Muir, Sierra Club Founder

Using my background in relaxation techniques and visualization as catalysts, while completing my doctorate I pursued training with many experts in the field, as well as advanced certification and approved supervisor status through the American Society of Clinical Hypnosis. This occurred during the years when these techniques were beginning to be used in medical settings, but were still out of the mainstream. Integrating these and other mind-body approaches into my clinical counseling practice seemed like a natural step for someone who had grown successfully through childhood cancer in part due to the unwitting personal employment of these techniques. If they had worked so well for me, I certainly wanted to be fully equipped to offer them to those I was assisting. In addition to using clinical hypnosis, visualization, and other relaxation approaches in medical and psychotherapeutic settings, I also became an instructor and supervisor of mental health professionals and physicians who were learning these invaluable tools. The approaches very effectively complemented my approach to counseling that included getting people into the great outdoors to explore all that nature holds, improving diet and exercise patterns, developing relationships, and engaging in enrichment activities.

The step to spending large amounts of time doing *pro bono* work with cancer and multiple sclerosis patients was a very natural one. As I thought back over the ways that I had dealt with my own cancer-related issues, there was an excitement about sharing this expertise with those in need. Escapes into what others called daydreams during my childhood were actually powerful self-induced visualizations that effectively assisted me in blocking pain, remaining comfortable during stressful situations, eliminating the horrors of nightmares, and inducing restful sleep. More often than not, these retreats involved detailed imagery of my beloved outdoor world with its plants and its animals. As a teenager, the same techniques helped me to cope with the residual effects of cancer, alleviate depression, deal with my father's death, and get on with my life in an easier fashion. Along the way, I also developed healthy diet and exercise patterns that teamed up with my life-long engagement with the natural world and its creatures to ensure my well-being.

Applying these and other cognitive-behavioral approaches across the board in my practice proved greatly beneficial to my patients. The Mayo Clinic provides a good definition of this common type of psychotherapy. "You work with a mental health counselor (psychotherapist or therapist) in a structured way, attending a limited number of sessions. Cognitive-behavioral therapy (CBT) can be a very helpful tool in treating mental health disorders, such as depression, post-traumatic stress disorder (PTSD), or an eating disorder. But not everyone who benefits from CBT has a mental health condition. It can be an effective tool to help anyone learn how to better manage stressful life situations."[3]

Often we can gain insight into ourselves and find crises easier to cope with through hearing the tales of those who have been in similar situations. It can be very helpful to read about how others have coped when faced with life challenges; how they have reached toward the natural world and its creatures; how they have used their experiences, memories, and imaginations to create a wealth of material for later use; how they have employed creative techniques to address their concerns; how they have found a healthier lifestyle; and how they have discovered alternative ways of bringing the natural world into their lives.

First, you will learn of my daughter's successful treatment for stage-three breast cancer and how she and I both made it though adversity. Then, I will share some of my own childhood cancer history and demonstrate how that experience and others evolved into gifts of insight into how to help others heal.

We will then look at two of the most common issues encountered when we are going through tough times: stress and sleep difficulties. I will also share several fabricated case studies that may help you move more comfortably through similar situations. Although case studies and descriptions of patient interactions are representative of my professional work, details have been dramatically altered and names are fictitional.

MAKING A DIFFERENCE
WHEN A LOVED ONE IS CHALLENGED

"In the depths of winter I finally found that there was within me an invincible summer." Albert Camus

Let's consider facing a challenge with a loved one. Can you think of a time when you felt unable to help as much as you wanted? Can you recall how out of control you felt when you wanted so much to be able to do something to make a difference? Can you remember how your own life was impacted? You might be in the throes of concern about a loved one's issues right now. A series of green space encounters and healthy physical and emotional investments can make a difference to your and your loved one's journey. Most of us have worried deeply about someone we love. Learning how my daughter and I got through one catastrophe may help you make your way through times when you are trying to help your family members or friends cope with crisis.

An enormous personal challenge came when my eldest daughter, Melissa, was threatened by stage-three breast cancer in her early thirties. Outdoor exercise in beloved green spaces, reaching out to others, tapping our inner resources, and staying deeply engaged in meaningful projects got Melissa and me through it—one day at a time. For her that also meant thirteen years of cutting-edge treatment and monitoring at Dana Farber Cancer Institute while completing her graduate work and then moving into a challenging, but rewarding, professional life as a Boston-based LICSW and LADC. Paralleling Melissa's engagements were my own body and soul-nurturing experiences and my volunteer work with environmental organizations. I followed the route to making a difference as I worked on behalf of Acadia National Park and the Maine coast. Those investments of time, energy, and dollars gave me the opportunity to act on behalf of the environment that has given me so much, while also helping me to instigate positive change during a time when I could not change what was happening for Melissa. Volunteerism itself is a healing tool during periods when the intrusions of illness, aging, or other issues prevent us from actively accessing the lands and waters that sustain us.

From its onset, parenting presents many twists and turns. We are not born knowing how to be the perfect parent. Unlike other warm-blooded creatures, we can't even count on basic mammalian instincts to carry us through. We muddle along, making the choices we think are best for our children, patching up the threat of damage from mistakes, and learning most of what we are doing along the way. What we do know is that the loving is instinctive. Much of the rest is a system of trial and error that we hope, in the end, produces an independently functioning and well-adjusted adult.

The majority of children in our society survive their childhoods despite their parents' mistakes. The greatest fear of most of the parents I know is that their children won't survive—that they will be stolen away by accident, disease, or some evil event. We do all we can to protect our children by helping them to make healthy choices that will keep them safe, giving them proper medical care and preventive treatments, and teaching them to take care of themselves in a sometimes-threatening world.

Occasionally, despite our best efforts, our children are threatened or taken from us. Other life challenges will also come our way, but these are two of the worst. Through sharing Melissa's and my experiences I offer companionship, coping skills, and hope to others who may be overwhelmed by challenges or a life crisis and to parents whose children are under attack. There is stress here on the word "coping." For, whatever life offers, we must go on—gathering up our inner resources, looking for the silver lining in the clouds, making lemonade out of lemons. And, while we are churning up the lemons for the lemonade, we can punctuate the chopping with visions of preserved spaces and experiences that can bolster us up for whatever is coming down the road. Some of the green space activities and related resources that Melissa and I used throughout her illness could find their way into your repertoire of healing techniques as well.

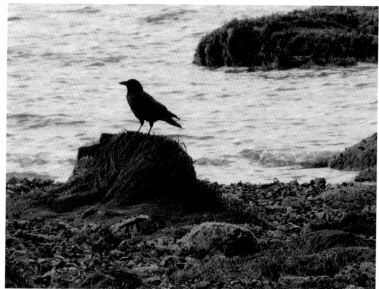

Melissa Savage

Crow on Critical Rockweed.

Melissa's Story

In the heart of Virgin Islands National Park, Little Lameshur Bay has extraordinary views of hillsides untainted by development. The only nighttime light other than the moon and the stars comes from a park ranger's cottage, a modest structure left over from the days when Laurance Rockefeller purchased the land for the park. Bordeaux Mountain rises above the bay, presenting an invigorating hike up the rocky trail where one may spot fat frangipani hornworms, golden orb spiders, and the elusive bridled quail dove.

Returning from one hike, Ben and I dove into the turquoise waters and snorkeled amidst the beautiful corals that lace the shores. Within minutes, the silversides arrived. Clouds of tiny, shining fish swam in schools thick as tapioca. From previous experience, we knew what we'd see next. Shooting directly at us came the first six-foot tarpon, followed by dozens more skimming by us like bullets. Caught up in the thrill of watching their feeding frenzy and knowing that they would turn away seconds before hitting us, we were shocked at suddenly being bombed from above. Brown pelican bills shot into the water all around us, frantically scooping up the silversides that the tarpon had driven to the surface. Flapping pelican feet paddled wildly as they swallowed their catch, their bills so full that the silversides spilled out by the hundreds. More bodies plummeted into the water, with slicked-back heads and beady little eyes creating a cartoon-like image. The boobies had joined us, greedily gobbling up the silversides as fast as they fell out of the pelicans' bills. Their appearance under water was so bizarre that we barely recognized these funny birds that we knew so well. For two hours or more, we swam with the silversides, tarpon, pelicans, and boobies, delighting in this most extraordinary experience. More than a decade later, this recalled experience fills me with delight and conjures up humorous images. I turn to it when I need a lift. There is a darker side of that memory, too. Little did I expect that shortly after this amusing snorkel, I would dive deeper emotionally than I had in a very long time. And, I would need every friend and every cognitive-behavioral approach I knew to make it through.

"Mummy, my new doctor wants me to have a mammogram." The words phoned from Maine to Virgin Islands National Park hit me like a bullet. Melissa, at age 33, had already had her share of medical problems. Before she was 30, severe endometriosis, fibroid tumors, and ovarian cysts had required a hysterectomy that left in its wake only one ovary. Two years before today's call, she had self-detected a breast lump and gone to her trusted physician in the state of alarm felt by all women in similar circumstances. Given her family history, we both expected she would be given a mammogram. Melissa's physician, opining that the lump was nothing to inspire concern, responded that at her young age there was no need for a mammogram. Fiction was created when the over-anxious mother was told that the mammogram had turned up nothing. A year went by, and then two. As she looks back on this situation, Melissa is protective of her physician, who she feels acted on her best instincts. I, on the other hand, feel outraged that my daughter's concerns about her body were ignored not once, but at two annual physicals when a palpable breast lump was present.

"I thought you'd had mammograms last year and the year before. What's going on?" I manage to croak.

"Well, I still have that lump and I didn't want you to be mad, but my old doctor didn't think I needed a mammogram." The onset of tears fills her voice. "I go in next week. Do you think I'm going to be okay?"

"Of course you're going to be okay. Only a very small percentage of breast lumps are a problem. There are so many different things that can crop up: cysts, fibroanenomas ...," I babble along in a convincing manner. Terrified myself, I try to sound calm, not wanting Melissa to experience that horrible limbo that comes with waiting for a diagnosis. And, indeed, there are many non-malignant, yet still worrisome, possibilities that shoot through my mind. Who would know better than Mummy, who had experienced them all?

My mind zooms to my own variety-fraught lump history, searching for more reassurance for Melissa. Before each of my own diagnoses, the prospect of "something else" threw me into a panic. How could my body, which I cared for so well, betray me? What would I do if the cancer was back after all these years? I had made it through college, marriage, graduate school, two babies, and combining this family of seven. Several lumps down the road as I lay on the examining room table, my doctor reported that he was finding a solid mass. I tried somewhat successfully to calm myself. Following my mind's eye to waving fan and tube corals, flitting blue chromis, and gliding angelfish, I immersed myself in the details of a snorkeling expedition. Once again, memories of a treasured experience took me to a better place. Leaving the hospital, I felt confidence return.

The nights between that day and when my biopsy results returned weren't so easy. Dreams of my father's rapid decline and death filled the darkest hours. My 2 AM terrors exploded with a huge sadness at the prospect of leaving my family and friends behind and of wasting away as my father had done. Childhood memories of Boston Children's Hospital loomed over my bed. Regardless of how composed I seemed during the day—moving from mental health patient appointments to meetings to parenting responsibilities to cleaning out the horse stalls—at night I had to really work to control my fears. I gathered up my inner resources, took my mind and my body to the green outdoors at every opportunity, and got myself under control. Each morning I raced along the carriage roads and across the trails of Acadia National Park, stopping at a special vista to thank God for giving me so much of life. I built stonewalls, adventured with Ben, divided and shared cherished plants, worked with the horses, fulfilled volunteer responsibilities, and talked with friends when I was not busy with patients or the family. I committed at least twenty minutes each day to a visualization and self-hypnosis exercise that incorporated imagery of Acadia or Virgin Islands National Park, knowing that would ease away some of the tension. Finally the report came back with a variety of abnormalities that led me down an eventful path.

Memories of that time are quickly replaced by the reality of Melissa's present crisis. In a matter of seconds, my mind has revisited another hell.

Talking with Melissa again later, I try to say the right things. "I know how scary this is, Liss, but it will most likely turn out to be nothing but a cyst or another kind of benign lump." My words stick in my throat as I pray silently, "Please don't let this happen to my child. If you need someone, take me instead." Trying not to sound panicked, yet wanting to stay in constant contact, I tell my dear eldest daughter that I will be calling her from our various anchorages over the next few days before our plane heads home.

Retreating further into my memories and my trusted method of visualizing my way to comfort, I create more distance from my current fears about Melissa's crisis as I close my eyes and do a progressive body relaxation exercise followed by some deepening techniques.

Visions surface of a crisp fall day's horseback adventure on Acadia National Park's magnificent Jordan Cliffs carriage road. We trot along, Liss and Beth babbling enthusiastically about Pony Club, anxious to tell Lib of the cross-country course in the latest event. Hundreds of feet of granite rise above us to the mountain's summit and plunge below to meet a sparkling blue Jordan Pond. The scent of decaying autumn leaves fills the air as hardwoods on the cliff face across the pond splatter the stands of evergreens with splashes of brilliant reds, golds, and oranges. The clip-clop of the horses' hooves along the gravel carriage road blends with our laughter and chatter as we soak in the splendor of the views and the ride.

Jordan Pond and the adjacent trails and carriage roads are stimulants for scores of memories in Acadia National Park, emphasizing the importance of this place in my life. From sparsely populated springs, we move to summers with the increased carriage road and trail use that the summer resident and tourist season brings. Families on rental bikes pedal past hikers who head for the Cliff Trail, the occasional reluctant participant hanging back from the group with the crankiest of expressions. The stream of cars pouring along the Park Loop Road is visible above the opposite shore. Each summer, scores of people head on foot, bike, by car or horse-drawn carriage toward the renowned Jordan Pond House for an afternoon of tea and popovers. Seated at birch tables on the sweeping lawns, the diners gaze across the pond to the little specks of our troop set against the drama of Jordan Cliffs on this blissful, innocent summer day.

My mind now floats to spring overlooking Acadia's Jordan Pond from the ledges above. The most delicate of greens breaks out in tiny leaf-buds covering the cliff faces with the promise of a new beginning. Some days bring muddy carriage roads with shards of frost still poking up through the earth and icicles dripping off the ledges. Other days the sun beats down on our faces, tricking us into thinking the cold weather has been left behind. No tourists here now, we have this place to ourselves on these early spring days.

Winter: shooting down the sloping carriage road on our cross country skis, skidding across the occasional ice patch, looking down upon frozen Jordan Pond at the thin strands of smoke blowing from the ice fishing shacks. We promise ourselves to try the skating later. It is a green wax day; cold air

fills our lungs as we speed along, looking forward to the next uphill, know-
ing it will warm our fingers and toes.

Another darkening winter afternoon, snowflakes coming down
with increased intensity, I arrive home to find a note from eight-year-
old Melissa taped to our kitchen table. "Dear Mummy, Chess and I
have skied to Jordan Pond. See you later! Love you, Lissy."

Lissy a capable skier, but eight. Chess, a beginner, at eleven. Dusk.
Ten degrees. The obvious route: the narrow, steep Asticou Trail. Numerous opportunities to drift off onto other trails. Panicked Mummy and
then Daddy call reliable skiing friends and all head off to find the girls.
Two hours later all return to Northeast Harbor with no girls. Pitch
dark. Five degrees. Snow coming down hard. I push open the snowy
kitchen door, shaking the snow from my hat, praying someone else
has found the girls. The warm glow of the lights produces Liss, Chess,
Bethy, and Granno all seated at the kitchen table cutting paper snowflakes, steaming hot chocolate with marshmallows and oatmeal cookies
in abundance.

"Where HAVE you been?" I sputter, overwhelmed with relief, joy,
and a fair bit of anger.

"We skied to Jordan Pond. I told you in the note," Melissa responds
smugly, her long damp hair and rosy cheeks enchanting me.

"How did you find your way back in the dark? You know you aren't
supposed to ski alone. Do you realize how cold it is? And it's dark.
Chessie doesn't even know how to ski. Do you realize what could have
happened? You are in BIG trouble!"

"But Mummy, you always say, 'Leave a note.' And I did. And I
taught Chess to ski. And I broke branches all along the trail so we
would know how to get back. And we're fine. Granno's here and we're
making snowflakes. You make one, too. And I made an angel outside in
the snow after I put my skis away. Let's go see if it's still there. I love you,
Mummy." My heart melts and I give in to relief and thanks for saving
my child one more time.

I contemplate many more Acadia memories as the promise of days
ahead glistens. And then I am back in the present where my children

no longer ride, or ski, or sail along in childhood innocence. They have come to know the adult world where, mingled with the delight and joy of life, are conflict, threats, and medical crises ready to jump out when one least expects them. How I wish I could protect them from these things. Sometimes I still manage to intervene, but today all I can do is join Melissa over the miles in her wait for her mammogram. Maybe I'm overreacting, imagining things, dwelling on the worst scenario. That is not like me. I'm so typically focused on the positive, ferreting out even the most difficult individual's attributes, finding that silver lining in every cloud. So why do I have this sick knot in the pit of my stomach right now, why am I waking up at 2 AM in a cold panic-sweat, why do I feel so certain that something is really wrong here?

Our friends, Lib and Frank, climb into the dinghy and Ben transports them through the choppy turquoise waters, depositing them at Customs where they will meet their ferry. Soon I will hear about Melissa's mammogram. Oh, please, let everything be all right. Tears well up in my eyes as I watch Ben and the dinghy, empty now of Lib and Frank and their bags, moving toward *Minerva* and pulling up alongside. Silently, I walk toward the lifeline gate, then turn on the cheer and begin chatting about the success of the visit. And it has been a good visit, despite my preoccupation with Melissa and her mammogram.

As we sail back to St. John, I think of our boatyard owner, Stu, and his wife, Paula. Little do I know that only a few short years later her own cancer will have returned and will be sapping her life away as all who love her stand by helplessly.

I go into a cleaning and packing frenzy, wanting to be sure everything is perfect before we head home for several weeks. Or am I just doing something that always makes me feel like I'm in control? Whenever the going gets tough, I start scrubbing regardless of how much else there is to do. We take off the jib and fold it into big flakes on the starboard deck. I stretch across the sail, extending my arms and legs as far as they will go, using my body as an anchor to hold down the sail in the stiff breeze. Ben folds again from the bow toward me, and we gather up the jib and stuff it neatly into the sail bag. Down the forward hatch it goes and we are ready for the next tasks.

Before we have even wound our way through Airport Security, laboring like Antiguan donkeys under our backpacks, I have mentally made the shift to our other life. In 54 hours, I will be home in my bed on Maine's Mount Desert Island for the first time in six weeks. I will have the added pleasure of recovering from the abdominal hernia surgery that will occur in 48 hours. By early in the following week Melissa should have received her mammogram results. Percentages remind me that all will likely be fine for her.

I pray for Melissa for a while and then throw in a prayer for myself, too. Despite the fact that I feel like a seasoned surgery veteran, I don't look forward to the experience, particularly the recuperation period that promises to foul up my outdoor activities for at least a couple of weeks. The jawbreaker-sized lump sticking out of my abdomen just above my navel reminds me that this surgery has been postponed as long as possible, however. Reassurance comes in the fact that I have so many times used a battery of resources that keep me as much engaged with the natural world as possible, even if I need to restrict athletic adventures. Writing, bird-watching, visual imagery, painting, gardening indoors or out, music, and volunteering on behalf of the environment can serve as tools to connect us in other ways with the green outdoors when we can't be our ideally active selves.

Thinking about my poor choice in lifting boulders until a hernia was produced, I ride the elevator up to my Boston hotel room, insert the key, and shove the door open. From across the darkened room I can see the red flasher on the phone.

Melissa's voice on the machine sounds tense. Within minutes she is on the line and speaking the words I had feared. "Mummy, they want me to have a biopsy tomorrow morning at 7:00 in Portland. The doctor is really worried. Can you meet me at the hospital?"

"Of course," I answer with my heart in my throat. We talk for a few more minutes until my shaking hand hangs up the phone. I hear the dial tone again and begin making arrangements to get to Portland, Maine. The fastest route is a car service that will pick me up at 3 AM. They will drive me to Mercy Hospital in what is something between a blinding blizzard and a freezing rainstorm. Slipping and sliding our way up the interstate, I hear the driver's tales of life and family. Assuming that my emergency departure from Boston had something to do with an ailing elderly relative, she is horrified to learn of my worries about Melissa. The driver has lost her sister to breast cancer just months ago. In her car, we bond and share our fears, despite the knowledge that we will likely never meet again.

At 7:10 AM, I climb out of the limo onto the icy hospital parking lot. The wind and snow whip around me as I slip my way toward the distant entrance, cursing the fact that I left my coat on the boat.

Then I remember that I also left my spare breast prostheses in the bathing suit that I had stuffed into the bag that would be delivered to the laundry. I could easily envision $600 worth of prostheses melting onto the inside of a hot dryer before our ferry had even made it to Charlotte Amalie. I could also imagine a puzzled laundry employee watching a prosthesis slip out of the laundry onto the floor as he or she was loading the machine. The humorous side of this broadened as I envisioned everyone in the Virgin Islands listening to Ben's blasting radio broadcast to Elite Laundry related to the endangered prosthesis.

No humor is with me now, however, as I hustle through the hospital to find Melissa and my sister, Lois. We barely have time to connect before the intake procedure begins. The surgeon, who has definitely avoided any medical school coursework in bedside manner, announces that, in addition to the palpable lump that Liss has been talking to her doctor about for two years, another one has been discovered in the mammogram.

Several hours later, a haze of appointments and tests behind her, Melissa is back at her house with her partner, Deborah. I am headed for Bangor, where Ben and I spend the night before my hernia surgery. Unable to eat because of my impending surgery, and unable to sleep due to my worries about Melissa, I stare into the darkness of the hotel room, talking to Ben about how much life seemed to have changed since we left the boat 36 hours ago.

By 5 AM, on Friday the 13th, I am filling out my own paperwork and telling anyone who will listen that just the day before I was with my daughter at Portland's Mercy Hospital. My friend and surgeon, Bill Horner, arrives and I pour out Melissa's story to him. Close to Melissa in his own right, he listens carefully in his patient manner and reassures me. Bill's thoughts cannot help but drift to the tragic loss of his wonderful son, Mark. A brilliant musician, rising star in the San Antonio Symphony, and a cherished friend of my daughter, Bethany, Mark had been brutally and senselessly murdered by a demented man in San Antonio not so long ago.

Bill reminds me that I am headed in for hernia surgery, something that I had always thought was reserved for men, and that I need to focus on that right now. I drift away in a fog of light anesthesia and follow my gray angelfish of self-hypnosis.

Smoothly, my body cuts through the surface of tranquil aqua waters, taking me to a place where I feel warm, comfortable, and bathed in the soothing liquid that surrounds me. Here I can be one with the fish, the corals, and the creatures of the sea. I can breathe deeply and normally as I join a school of iridescent blue chromis, drifting in and out of gaps in the corals. The gentle motion of the sea moves us back and forth, back and forth, as we feed upon the corals, gaining sustenance and strength. Appearing out of the deeper blue waters is another beauty of the sea, the gray angelfish. We follow and go deeper, closely watching her movement, observing each detail of her body. She moves with the current and the sea, effortlessly, as do we. Her body is a large, gray disc with light-edged dark scales. Delicate fins assist in moving her forward. I notice that her tail is cut square and that her pectoral fins show yellow. She has a white snout and her up-turned lips are lined darker. She guides us deeper into the corals, into a safe, comfortable, and relaxed place where we can rest and restore ourselves as we drift deeper and deeper. Later, we will awake feeling refreshed, relaxed, with renewed energy, with no stiffness, numbness, or heaviness in any part of our body, knowing that we can return to this very pleasant place under the sea whenever we desire…simply by closing our eyes and moving down, down through the warm aqua waters to swim freely with the fish. Every moment is a soothing, healing, and strengthening experience. For now we just go deeper and deeper still, feeling more and more relaxed…

A few hours later, Ben packs my repaired hernia and me into the car for the hour's drive home. The only hitch is that I am not quite ready to go. Something good needs to be wedged into these wretched two-and-a-half days. I insist that we drive an hour or so out of our way to a Christmas tree farm. He suggests that, if we do, I need to choose the tree from the car. That is not the way I do things. At a right angle and clutching my stomach, I emerge from the car and trudge up and down the rows of trees looking not for just one perfect tree but for three. I like to have them everywhere, their little white lights reflecting throughout the house, covered with all the decorations from years and generations past.

Happy to have my trees and headed home after weeks away, I monologue to Ben about Melissa and the events of the past two days as we drive toward Mount Desert. Jerking to alertness and reaching too far to grab the ringing cell phone, I yelp in pain. "Mummy, how was your surgery? Oh, Mummy, I have cancer. Can you come back down on Monday and go to the doctor's with me?

"No, Mummy, don't come sooner. You need to rest from your surgery." I reel with the uncertainty of what comes next, what power rests in the words of physicians, and how helpless we can feel in the face of challenge. Shaking my head to expel the images, I take a huge breath and consider how I can begin to mobilize my inner resources, gather up the knowledge from a lifetime of refining crisis management skills, and begin to march forward on my daughter's behalf. It feels like I am about to go to war. But, I know that whatever lies ahead, there are ways to make it easier and increase the odds.

I am a fixer of things, from pets to nonprofits to gardens to people, but I am terrified that I cannot fix this. Steeling myself against the greatest dread, I begin to analyze the threads that can be woven together to create a carefully-crafted approach to psychological survival during a period of extreme crisis. Those thoughts begin to crystallize:

Seek out family and friends, share your feelings, and strengthen your support team.

Look at who else is in the circle of care and incorporate them and their expertise into the team.

Activate cognitive-behavioral strategies, choosing activities that will strengthen the mind, the body, and the spirit.

Engage with the natural world as actively as possible to get the endorphins going and build up as much positive energy as possible.

Seek out the natural world and its creatures for relaxation, solace, and immersion in beauty.

Express thanks for the good things.

Use relaxation techniques and creative visualization regularly to relieve fatigue and stress and to enhance a host of other issues from positive focus to recovery from surgery.

Choose healthy eating habits, using food as fuel.

Bring as much beauty as possible into life through the arts and the intersection of art and nature.

Give back to the world in some meaningful way. There is a place to make a difference, even when some aspects of life feel out of control.

I know that each of these things will help me to be stronger for Melissa and that she also will seek out these resources. So many times throughout life they have helped me to push through difficult times. So many times I have seen them help to heal my patients, family members, friends, and professional peers. Please let them work effectively this time as well.

Spinning downward, I make a plan to meet Melissa in Portland on Monday, December 16, 2002, for what will turn out to be a series of medical appointments. Recovery from my hernia surgery is put on the back burner. For the weekend, I continue walking tenderly around at a right angle as I pack my bag again, fill the car with gas, and host an impromptu Saturday night distraction dinner. We dine informally in our living room, talking about conservation, Afghani women's interests, and Melissa. Attempting at some humor, we laugh about a carefree evening when, at Friends of Acadia's gala to benefit projects at Acadia National Park, several of us named Diana/Dianna offered ourselves up as caterers for a dinner in our artist friend, Richard Estes', dining room. Taking a risk that no one would "buy" us, and with a sense of humor, we made a difference to some green space in the natural world with a good winning bid. Jolting back to the present, I think once more of what I might do to make a difference somewhere when I can do so little to change the course of my daughter's life.

I am raw and emotional, my thoughts flitting constantly to what Melissa and Deborah must be experiencing this weekend. Instead of a relaxing break filled with their favorite outdoor activities, they are beginning a terrifying and threatening journey.

I-95 seems like a rocky, potholed back road to my wounded belly as I wince my way through the three-hour drive, arriving at the hospital in time to join Melissa for her consultation. She has already met this doctor and is not impressed, put off by pushiness and too much expression of alarm and negativity. The karma is clearly not good. My reaction is similar, but we put the surgeon's recommendations on our calendars: immediate mastectomy followed by chemotherapy and radiation. Melissa wants to be treated in Portland. She does not want to miss any classes or work. Period. Numbly, we leave the hospital and talk about getting together again later in the week. Melissa returns to work.

I begin the drive home, allowing my internal autopilot to take the exit that heads me for the Maine Coast Heritage Trust office, a place where I might be able to help to make a difference during this tumultuous time. Opening the door a crack, then wider, I slip into our Campaign for the Coast meeting.

Richard Rockefeller, our leader, and his small committee greet me with surprise, having been told that I had not intended to make this meeting due to my hernia surgery. I cave in, break down, and tell them of the recent events with Melissa. We proceed with our meeting. These good friends are clearly jarred by what I have told them. I am trying to hold it together, knowing that life over the coming months must continue despite this terrible addition to it. Richard pulls me aside during our break and we arrange to meet later to talk about the crisis. Melissa's crisis. My crisis.

Richard is in the midst of his own crisis and knows well the rollercoaster ride that a cancer patient experiences. A highly respected physician and nonprofit volunteer, he has been in the throes of his own cancer for months. He meets my traumatized gaze and asks me what plans have been made for Melissa's treatment. I share the plan and tell him of our discomfort with the surgeon, as well as Melissa's intention to be treated in Portland. He firmly suggests that this is a time when, for Melissa's well-being, I must insist that she get a second opinion at Dana Farber where they are approaching advanced stage estrogen-receptive breast cancer in a whole new way. Little do I know that this talented, caring friend has given us a direction that will save Melissa's life or that he, years later, will be snatched away from all who love him by a tragic accident.

Family and friends weave the fabric that is life. When we are happy or in crisis we regularly connect with one another. Verbalizing our feelings is not a problem for most of those in my closest relationship circle. This time is different. Somehow it seems that if I don't speak the words, this won't be real.

My caretaker-self tells me that if I don't seek out those I love, I will be swallowed up by grief. I pick up the phone and begin pushing the numbers. Hours later, I have talked to twenty or thirty friends and I am still not through. I postpone my summer friends, except for Ruth and

Tris, who offer just the right thoughts, hoping to have some encouraging words before I reach out to others across the miles. At the end of the day, I have a sense of being recharged. Although the situation is indeed more real, my friends' words of encouragement and caring, their stories of those who have made it through the worst kinds of cancer, and their unconditional love have helped me to replenish my supply of energy and optimism.

When they ask me what they can do to help, I tell them Melissa might like a note and prayers. And I say, "Please tell me the good things that are happening in your life. I need to hear about the things that are making you happy." As they share their joy, I smile through my tears and thank God for bringing each of these wonderful people into my life.

Melissa's treatment at Dana Farber is a world away from what she would have received closer to home. Herceptin and careful monitoring by her oncologist, Dr. Eric Weiner, see her through the early stages of her treatment. The Herceptin and other drugs do their jobs and she moves through surgery with tumors of reduced size. Chemotherapy becomes part of Melissa's life and mine as we ride the bus together to Dana Farber.

Many visits to Dana Farber later, a brown-cushioned seat awaits me across from the nurse's station, one of many ringing a series of horse-shoe-shaped waiting areas throughout the hospital. I know the routine now and head to the snack table for a couple of waters while Melissa checks in. Settling into the chair, I glance surreptitiously toward the room's corner where an anxious sixtyish woman sits twisting her tissue into knots while her husband absorbs the last of *The Wall Street Journal*. She whispers, he nods, not looking up, and goes back to his paper. A tear falls from the corner of her eye and rolls down her crinkled cheek as she catches it with the wadded tissue. Biting her lip, she reaches for her husband's hand as he pulls away and turns another *Journal* page. Tears begin flowing more freely while she stuffs her hand into a black leather shoulder bag and rummages for more tissues.

Melissa turns from the nurses' station, assesses the situation, and walks casually toward the woman, offering a box of tissues and a smile. Her bald head announces that she is ahead of the woman in this game. She moves toward me, accepts a water bottle, pulls a statistics book from her backpack, and settles in again to wait.

The arrival of Melissa's art therapist takes her away to another space where they will talk and paint for the next hour. A natural artist who drifts in and out of watercoloring, throwing pots, and painting occasional oils, Melissa finds this Dana Farber water coloring offering is a welcome retreat. From my own work with cancer patients, I know how helpful artistic expression can be for those who are longing to release their emotions as well as for those who are just seeking a change of focus for a while.

My mind flits to the fact that this art therapist, like Melissa, is a graduate student. Like the young divinity school student who offers her calming demeanor to Melissa and the other patients each time they are here. Like the serious residents and interns who are putting in their twenty hours a day and have not yet learned not to wear their hearts on their sleeves. Like Melissa, who studies and prepares for exams while waiting for chemotherapy, makes the long trip home fighting off stomach discomfort the whole way, and sees her own clients at the refugee re-settlement program the next morning.

How does she do it, this combining of illness, treatment, worrying, studying, planning, working, and giving to others in her own internship? And why, of all the busy graduate students around her, is she the one coping with cancer? I bite my own lip now and glance up to see the woman in the corner sending a hesitant smile in my direction. "Your daughter?" she asks. I nod and return her smile. "She's beautiful," she says, and I know she is speaking not just of Melissa's physical beauty, but also of her spirit and the way she reaches out to others. We make our way through the day, this beautiful daughter of mine and I, returning later to our respective homes to await the next dawn.

3:30 came early this morning. For years, I have delighted in the pre-dawn hours—bustling about the house preparing for the day ahead; nestling into the sofa pillows with a good book, a steaming mug of Earl Grey tea, and our fluffy kitty; or zipping out the door with a head lamp on my way for a solitary Acadia run.

Today is different. My eyes fly open as I hear, "…some bone scans…not good…not good…not good…"

Dreaming. Those weren't real words. But, it is all somehow real. Melissa. The bone scan. That part was okay. Calm down. You are here in your warm bed nestled up against Ben's backside, his low snoring the only sound in the room. Melissa is in Boston with Deborah, enjoying a long weekend. Bethany is stuck in a blizzard on her way to Baltimore. Everyone is okay. No, wait, everyone is not okay. Bethany and Kristin and Thor and Chafee and so many others are fine. But, Melissa is not. It is 3:45. I climb out of bed and creep out to our dark office to turn up the heat. In the kitchen, Mickey's yowl for breakfast and pats is something I can count on.

To break the pattern of fear, I contemplate the emerging dawn and begin to write a visualization script that conjures up images of St. John and Virgin Islands National Park—a place Melissa and I both adore. Perhaps you would like to use parts of this script to transport yourself to the protected lands and waters of Virgin Islands National Park. You can record it or have someone read it to you.

Our eyes gently close and we begin breathing freely and deeply, freely and easily, drifting down, down to a more and more relaxed place. Amidst bursts of azures, turquoises, and greens, our journey begins on the tropic isle of St. John, home of the Virgin Islands National Park. We wind our way to Little Lameshur Bay, a perfect pearl on the necklace of enchanting harbors ringing this lovely island. Sugar sand, sparkling waters, and a gentle, warm, and caressing breeze whisper promises of time beneath the sea, but first we will explore the miracle of the land base between here and Reef Bay, whose sugar mill ruins speak to a time when things were not so easy on St. John. Paying respect to those who toiled, we turn toward the canopy of tamarind trees and follow the winding Lameshur trail, confident that there will be delight at every turn. The melodic notes of the pearly-eyed thrasher pierce the silence as a flock of smooth-billed ani call out a greeting chorus. We breathe deeply of the scent of sage mingled with that of the wet, steamy earth. Little hermit crabs housed in seashells roll their way down the slope, gathering up in family parties here and there. These creatures, ranging from barely visible to baseball-sized, reside in abandoned shells and move to larger accommodations as they grow. On this day, following a nurturing rain, the mud squishes underfoot, belying the existence of many cacti amidst the thick growth. Ahead, a blizzard of great southern white and sulfur butterflies explodes, tempting closer examination. One rests upon a branch, offering the opportunity to view its delicate translucent wings and turquoise-tipped antennae. Dozens of these white and pale yellow fairies hover over the vegetation waiting to plunge their proboscis deep into the throats of flower hosts to advance the pollination process. Flitting about, they transport the pollen from blossom to blossom, sometimes gathering to sip and extract minerals from wet areas in a process called "puddling." We settle down amidst their fluttering to contemplate the miracle of their procreation. As many as 500 tiny torpedo-shaped eggs are attached by each female to the leaves of the timber caper tree. If this can happen in nature, there are all sorts of possibilities for us. Miracles can happen. Dark-haired, black-spotted caterpillars sporting yellow back-stripes later emerge from the eggs, growing and feeding hungrily on the succulent leaves over the next two to three weeks. Bursting with energy, each caterpillar transforms itself into a hard-shelled chrysalis and, seven days later, each chrysalis opens to reveal a young butterfly ready to perpetuate the cycle of the great southern white. Another miracle.

Ahead, a ferret-like mongoose darts past us, likely headed for a raid on one more bird's nest. Transported to the Eastern Caribbean from India to feed upon the islands' rats, the growing population of mongoose has finished off many rats and now works on decimating the island's avian residents. They are interesting creatures, however, conjuring up images of Kipling's Riki Tiki Tavi, which sheds a softer light upon them.

As the trail climbs, becoming more rock-strewn, views of Reef Bay stretch ahead, its sparkling waters and inviting cove promising exquisite snorkeling. The climb behind us, our bodies welcome the downhill trek back into a canopy of tangled vegetation. A flash of orange, yellow, and black alerts us to a frangipani hornworm laboring its way across the trail. Thrilled, we scooch down to get a closer look at this dashing, plump clown of a caterpillar. He rears up slightly, appearing to examine us, and then humps along his way with his bright reddish orange head taking the lead as it sways from side to side determining a course. There once was a woman who so treasured her garden that she sprayed poisons upon these fantastic creatures rather than share her blossoms with them. The message for us is, "Learn to share the world and live in harmony with its precious creatures." Meanwhile, the frangipani's time is short in his garish caterpillar garb, and he is destined for a stint as a rather mundane-looking giant gray sphinx moth.

We detour and trek to The Petroglyphs, a spiritual place where time stands still. Water cascades down a sharp cliff face to fall in tranquil pools below. Delicate red dragonflies dart across the water's surface through shafts of filtered sunlight. We sit awhile by this healing pool and let the elements of the spirit seep deep into our bodies and our minds, healing us and strengthening us from within. High above, huge trees stretch up to meet the sky. Scrambling up the crumbling hillside through the thorny brush, we reach the top and gaze down upon a series of waterfalls, pools, and dragonflies to the place where petroglyphs are etched upon the stone. "Who came here to scratch upon the wall so many years ago and how many generations of different types of people have seen this place?" we wonder. We pay homage to all who have come before us and give thanks for the opportunity to be a part of this wondrous world, praying for healing as we go.

After The Petroglyphs, we hike up another side spur to the Mexican creeper-covered Reef Bay Great House. The vines' bright pink flowers grow in great profusion, climbing readily over fences, trees, and stone houses across the Eastern Caribbean. A treat awaits us as, in awe, we approach the Great House. Swarms of honeybees, butterflies, hummingbird bees, wasps, and other such creatures feast upon the stunning blossoms of the vine, creating a steady hum of pleasure at the abundance of nectar. They accept our careful study of their distinguishing markings and focus on their business, seemingly oblivious to our presence. Skirting along a side trail that leads to the ruins of the Danish landlords' slave quarters, we again contemplate the importance of learning to live in harmony with one's neighbors, whether humans, bees, or other creatures. Our role as stewards of this world extends to the caretaking of others through kindness and an absence of exploitation.

Bushwhacking through the pointed sansevera, we again join the Reef Bay trail, hike to the sugar mill ruins, follow the L'Esperance trail to the top, and climb the paved road to the Bordeaux Mountain trail. We find ourselves in cooler, fresher air at this height, breathe it in, and restore ourselves. A clump of tropic milkweed—orange and pink Asclepias—draws us to the sheer delight of watching dozens of butterflies feeding upon it—sulfurs, Southern whites, fritillaries, zebras, and the joyful presence of four endangered monarchs. Spellbound, we reflect on their journey from the northeast and reconfirm our thoughts that, if butterflies and birds can persevere year after year in their migration, we can take on any challenge. We then recall a time on Maine's protected Brimstone Island where, one sparkling autumn day, we found ourselves amidst thousands of monarchs. There to feed upon the common milkweed form of Asclepias on their trip south, they were inclined to land on our heads, arms, and other body parts as if we were just one more milkweed. Now the monarchs struggle to survive as their critical stopovers are deforested and stripped of the vegetation that nourishes them. What joy there is in discovering four of these orange and black striped beauties while on our tropic adventure. What can we do to promote their survival? Plant milkweeds! Encourage the native, somewhat invasive variety in the northeast and nurture the tropic annual Asclepias in our seasonal garden. And, we will plant a spiritual milkweed for ourselves and our loved ones so that it is there to feed and nourish our bodies and our souls with each breath that we take, with each word that we speak. Healing, soothing, restoring, and relaxing.

Images of Maine monarchs merge into St. John visions and the trip down the vegetation-lined Bordeaux Mountain trail. Ahead, a bridled quail dove tucks itself shyly into the bushes, bobbing its head and tail as it goes. This secretive bird is a rare sighting, in contrast to the more common doves of St. John, and we are thrilled at its presence. We leave it to return to its fragile, spindly nest high up in the branches as we pick our way down the mountain trail, stepping carefully around numerous rolling hermit crabs. The expansive view of Caribbean waters stretches ahead with Little Lameshur Bay, our return destination, beckoning. We rest here a little while longer and, when we are ready, we open our eyes feeling very, very good throughout, relaxed, yet refreshed with renewed energy.

Throughout her medical challenge, Melissa employed a variety of healing techniques, to augment her care. These included visualization, massage, acupuncture, meditation, and group therapy. When she could, she ran, biked and swam. She painted, potted, and threw clay on the wheel. She reached out to others time and again and helped them to heal. Here is another visualization connected to the waters that she loves—this one with some fun and additional messages.

"I'd like to be, under the sea, in an octopus's garden in the sun," we sing happily through our snorkels, our memories, or our imagination. And, what a garden it is. Beneath the silken surface of the undulating sea lies a vast plane for exploration. Our strong arms and legs take us over the sparkling sand and though the aqua waters toward the reefs that ring St. John's Waterlemon Cay anchorage. Movement in the sand reveals a pointed tail and two bulbous eyes that stick up through the sand. A few flips and a juvenile southern stingray reveals itself. With a body only five or six inches long, he is truly a baby. We parallel his path and hover over as he settles in once more, this time attracting a host of fish who begin to clean his body. In apparent ecstasy, he lifts one side and then the other, allowing the "cleaner fish" the opportunity to give him a very thorough scrub. What a symbiotic relationship they have, these industrious cleaners and those whose bodies they feed upon. A larger cleaner fish than these, the remora, with its suction cup head, can attach itself to its host turtle or ray and ride along while also feeding. Our baby ray, well-cleaned, gracefully glides away while we turn our attention to an abundant school of deep blue tangs. The tangs move slowly in a group with one trumpet fish ensconced amidst the school, looking like a wanna-be tang.

We anthropomorphize the creatures of this sea that binds us all together as it flows from the enticing waters of the Virgin Islands National Park to the icy shores of Acadia and far, far beyond. The smiling and gregarious blue tangs remind us of those happy souls who go about their business, threatening no one, chit-chatting constantly and making new friends. As they drift effortlessly past a gang of yellow and black striped sergeant majors, the furious sergeants bolt toward us and the tangs, appearing angry, or perhaps just insecure, as we invade their territory. Excitement builds as a ponderous hawksbill turtle paddles by while he munches casually at vegetation. Two remoras hitch a ride upon his back—traveling, without cost, to parts unknown. Many folks like a free ride, too, regardless of the destination. Oh, flashy and beautiful stoplight parrot fish, dressed in colors of blue, green, pink, and yellow, should we take the time to seek your substance below the surface, or just enjoy the view? And how about you? Do you swim through life, assuming that your beauty will get you by, forgetting that old age could find you colorless? Or, do you use that beauty to help you to improve the world, attracting others to your cause, inspiring hope, building up your inner beauty?

A multitude of fish surround us, cheery black and white spotted trunkfish, a big-lipped margate, scores of snappers, wrasses of every hue, blue runners steaming by, more rays and turtles, all thriving in this lovely place with corals waving and welcoming all around. There they are: fat fish, skinny fish, red fish, blue fish, Christian fish, Jewfish, gay fish, straight fish, boisterous fish, shy fish, all living in seeming harmony. Perhaps our world can learn something from theirs.

What could be more thrilling than swimming along above a ten-foot-wide spotted eagle ray? The defined head of the eagle ray looks nearly human with its watchful eyes and long, bulbous nose. It gracefully flaps its wide, spotted wings, stirring up delicacies with its nose. The thrill is enhanced ten-fold as we are blessed with the presence of the eagle ray's three-foot-wide little one, who soars in to dig some dinner. We hover patiently above, here in Leinster Bay on St. John, then swim along, entranced by the feeding eagle rays and feeling so privileged to a part of their world. Ahead lies Waterlemon Cay, a jewel of a little island surrounded by magnificent corals that feed a host of fish. A strip of glistening sand binds the sea to this rocky outcropping of an island, stretching into the watery home of an abundance of rays, turtles, and reef fish that feed and live among magnificent corals. Swimming steadily toward the outside of Waterlemon, paralleling Sir Frances Drake channel, we glide smoothly over dozens of isolated coral heads. Blue parrot fish drift by, followed by a school of juvenile stoplight parrot fish. A flash of black and white catches our attention, and we spot one of our favorites, a spotted trunkfish. This comical little fish with his turned-up snout and propeller fins is always a delight. This time there are two spotted trunks, outlined against a waving purple fan coral and joined by a plump and smiling balloon fish. Looking like a happy porcupine with his spiny body, the balloon fish is quick to duck into a cave and then peek shyly out. Look him in the eye and he will give you a smile that stretches all the way across his face. Flitting in and out amongst the coral garden are a host of bright-colored wrasses: blueheads, yellowheads, and the occasional slippery dick. Reluctant groupers sidle up closely to rocks and corals, seeming to nearly take the shape of their protector, and slip into holes when approached. And, of course, tucked around most coral heads are a multitude of squirrelfish, sergeant majors, parrots of various types, and many babies of a wide variety. The babies and the budding young corals whisper what may be false promises of a future during this time of rapid environmental change, but we take heart in what we see, recalling a partial recovery from the vast coral bleaching of a few years ago. Our expedition is a great success, as we feel ourselves becoming one with the ocean, the waving corals, and the scores of sea creatures. We slow our swim to float gently along on the waves, rolling to look up at the sky above. The waters that bind us all together, the limitless sky stretching out to zones unknown, and the protected lands of this unique and special shoreline fill us with a sense of awe and overwhelming appreciation for all that we behold. We pledge to do what we can to help to care for this world and her creatures, knowing that we are one with them and realizing that we can bring back in our mind's eye, whenever we choose, the details of every aspect of this place at this point in time. The waters upon which we drift along soothe and heal us, nurturing our body and our soul, penetrating our very being with their strengthening and healing potential. We emerge when we are ready, feeling warm and comfortable, stronger and healthier, confident and optimistic, looking forward to each new day, feeling very, very good throughout. And, whenever we choose, we can close our eyes and drift right down again to this very place, joining the creatures, the corals, the sea for another healing experience.

This is how you begin to create a visualization script. You might like to try your hand at it now. Whatever happens is just fine. Just relax and let yourself go.

Write a detailed description that will draw you into a special place. If you choose, precede your visualization with the progressive relaxation script in Chapter Three of this book. Include other messages that are meaningful to you, will inspire change, and present opportunity for exploration. Record your script or ask someone to read it to you while you rest comfortably, with your eyes closed. It helped us during a trying time and I hope it helps you, too.

Melissa fared well in the first phase of her treatment and busily pursued her graduate studies, missing not one class. As her hair grew in, she ran

a half marathon and biked the Pan Mass Challenge with her Dana Farber oncologist, Dr. Eric Weiner. She painted and played with friends,
enjoyed her puppy, and went off with Deborah to explore the great
outdoors at every available opportunity. We all tried to get back to some
semblance of normal, although the threat of cancer was ever-present.

"Hi there, Liss. Just checking in. Hope you had fun in Province-
town and a good dinner with your friends. Tomorrow we leave Bequia
headed for Dominica. It's about a thirty hour sail in this wind, so I want
to catch up with you today." Trying not to sound nervous. Needing to
know where things stand. "I'll try you back in a little while."

I join our sailing buddy, Clare Shepley, and Ben on deck for a final
look at the stars. They both know I am terrified. Clare heads forward to
her guest quarters. Ben and I climb into our aft cabin bunk and, amaz-
ingly, I sleep until 4 AM.

In the early dawn light, we make the final preparations for departure. Clare stows loose objects, and Ben begins to get the anchor up as
I tack back and forth to set it free. We sail slowly out of the Bequian
anchorage, round the comer into the morning breeze, and set our course
for St. Vincent where we plan to have one more snorkel before heading
offshore. Ben streams the fishing line with its new pink Bequian lure
as we all joke about our marginal fishing skills. I, in particular, am not
a fisherman, preferring to think of the fish swimming freely instead.
With some reluctance I admit fresh fish taste a lot better than those
from packages, and I join the fray.

Within an hour we see the boiling evidence of blackfin tuna
schooling on the water's surface and soon get a strike. Ben reels in the
thrashing fish and hooks it with the gaff while Clare prepares to give
it a shot of whiskey in the gill to bring on death quickly. We thank the
ocean for her gift.

The promise of fresh sushi is too much to resist. As quickly as Ben
cuts the fish into steaks for the next few dinners, Clare scoops the scraps
up off the deck and savors their delicious freshness. Tall, sophisticated,
and beautiful, Clare is not the sort one would expect to indulge in this
kind of behavior. I turn from the wheel, grab the camera and take what
will be one of our more memorable photos of her. Then I put the boat

on autopilot and join her for what proves to be a great treat.

Morning sunlight pours over *Minerva's* decks and the waters around us as we slip into a quiet St. Vincentian cove and one of the most beautiful Caribbean anchorages we know. Over the side we go, marveling at the steep, palm-covered hillside above us and the extraordinary corals that lie below. I immerse myself in the beauty under the water's surface. Schools of blue chromis and tangs drift by, joined by brilliant parrot fish, rock beauties, and French angels. The corals are some of the most incredible I have ever seen and I easily lose myself in the search for hiding morays and octopus. Snorkeling is such a healing experience for me—the place I retreat to in my dreams and visualizations. This time I am rewarded with an octopus sighting. He sits peering warily out of his cave, turning blue when I approach to get a closer look. I could stay here forever. Ben and Clare join me in my find and we delight in this rare experience. Reluctantly, we swim back to the boat looking forward to the passage ahead, but sorry not to have more time in this bit of paradise.

Tucking into my sea bunk before dark, I know I have six hours to sleep until my 2 AM watch. Clare is settled into her watch, harnessed into the cockpit, enjoying the last of the twilight. Ben checks our course, turns on our running lights and lies down until his watch begins at 11:00. I thank God for the world and her creatures, these two dear people, my many other friends and family, and I pray for their well-being. A special plea is for Melissa and a good recovery. I drift away, like a speck on the sea, wake spontaneously at 1:50, pull on my gear, and meet Ben on deck. He gives me a loving pat, updates me on our course, traffic and weather, and goes below for some sleep. My night watch is the kind we all wait for. The boat sails smoothly through the swells, pushed along by a 15-knot breeze. The Southern Cross is a wonderful sight. Tears splash down my face as I consider its beauty and what specks of insignificance we humans are in comparison. The loom of the lights of Martinique beckon to a parade of four cruise ships making their way south for a morning arrival. Their passengers are full of wine and heavy food, I trust, sleeping soundly through this lovely night in preparation for a day of beaches and shopping ashore.

Recalling other close encounters, I hope their captains are alert and aware that they share the sea with us.

It is a night of long, low seas. A sailboat's lights are running parallel to port, perhaps also bound for Dominica. I speculate on who might be aboard and what their stories might be. We all do have our stories. They are punctuated by the intense highs and lows of personal achievements and challenges, family milestones, weddings, babies, illnesses, and funerals. They are colored by the ebb and flow of the years in between. A common thread runs through for most of us: the depth of caring that we have for at least one other person or living thing and the despair we feel when that loved one is threatened or lost. The other sailboat's cabin lights come on and twinkle across the sea, inviting me to feel a bond with those aboard. In some way, I know that my story is not so different from theirs.

A sense of comfort sweeps over me as I sail along through the night. What a relief it is to have this respite from worry. The sea is the place where I am most at home, where Ben and I are at our best. We have sailed thousands of miles together over the years, ninety percent of the time with no one else aboard. The ease of interaction, the appreciation of the world around us, and our shared interests make this such an important part of our existence. It enables us to effectively meet the challenges of the rest of life. Despite my worries, I am able to relax in the motion of the boat, focusing on all my blessings. A rosy glow peeks through the piled-up pillows of early morning clouds, exposing the breaking dawn. Shafts of sunlight make false promises of a fine day, and a red sun rises.

So, there you have a taste of my tale of a loved one faced by challenges. The relief still floods over me when I write that, over fourteen years after her diagnosis, Melissa is healthy and flourishing. After many long years of experimental treatments and monitoring, her oncologist, Dr. Eric Weiner, announced that she was essentially cured. She is a licensed clinical social worker (LICSW) working in a medical setting in Boston, helping patients with their own sets of issues. My heart swells with pride at her generous-spirited nature and the woman that she has become.

I hope that the route to integrating healthy approaches while dealing with life challenges, or implementing them when things are just fine, is becoming clearer. Sometimes the challenging times can seem insurmountable, but you can get there.

Take a moment to think again about your own situation. You could make some notes, write freely, or tape a recording of your story. Note your current situation or your challenge and its nature: personal medical issue; crisis with a loved one; work or responsibility-related problem; or issues connected to aging. List the ways in which you are being impacted and the areas you want to work on. If you want, you can use Melissa's and my crisis as an example. Beyond mobilizing a support team, employing relaxation techniques and creative visualization, and drawing upon memories of great adventures in the natural world, there are a number of other techniques that Melissa and I both used throughout the course of her illness. These can help to smooth the path when we are stressed, worn out, overwhelmed by work and responsibilities, or slowed down by accident, illness, or the aging process. And, they can all be used as preventive medicine to help every one of us to keep functioning at an optimal level. They include:

Clean up your diet and beverage consumption, cutting back or eliminating alcohol, sugar, and caffeine. If nicotine is a part of your life, get that out, too.

Engage in the green outdoors at every opportunity.

Practice relaxation techniques and visualization, incorporating memories and images of the natural world and her creatures.

Give thanks daily for the good things in your life.

Reach out in a positive way to at least one other living thing each day.

Exercise at whatever level works for you, outdoors if possible.

Interact frequently with family, friends, and other living creatures.

Express yourself in a creative manner. Paint, write, arrange flowers, or whatever strikes your fancy.

Find humor.

Engage in a volunteer experience where you can make a difference.

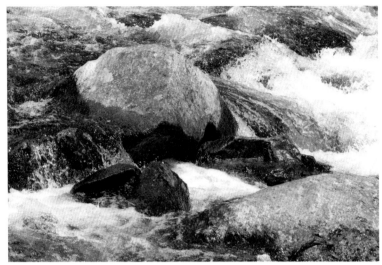

Sheridan Steele

You Can Calm Life's Turbulent Waters.

DIARIES AND MEMORIES: PART I

MOVING PAST CHILDHOOD CANCER THROUGH VISUALIZATION AND ENGAGEMENT WITH NATURE

"The best environmental stewardship is intergenerational, because early childhood impressions are imprinted so strongly and absorbed so deeply."
Aaron Mair, Sierra Club President

The coping mechanisms that even a young child can develop on his or her own can be as effective as professionally-prepared approaches to direct engagement with the natural world and other healthy lifestyle elements. The outdoor activities and living creatures to which a little child and others gravitate, and the replacements for those when they are not available, are natural relievers of stress, anxiety, feelings of lack of control, and a sense of being overwhelmed.

As you read the inner thoughts of a young girl as she grows, I hope that you will see how green space adventures, alternative healing techniques, and related activities can push any of us through tough times. I was this child and I made it. For that, many credits are due: to our world and her creatures, to my relatives and friends, to a remarkable series of medical professionals, to a healthy lifestyle, to a host of excellent volunteer engagements, to good fortune and good education, to an appreciation of each moment of every day, and to God and our Universe. Thank you.

You also can make it through the challenges that life presents while marching on to a time when you can bring all of what is offered back to assist you throughout life and the aging process. Here is a bit about how it all began for me and how childhood traumatic illness served as the catalyst and inspiration for the creation of healing experiences. I hope you will see the potential for yourself in what I share of my own history and my professional work. Spontaneously integrating the healing power of the natural world and related techniques into my life helped me survive the trauma of childhood cancer and other life stressors. These techniques ultimately helped my patients, friends, and family members as well. It is likely that you will identify with some of these challenges. You are welcome to make these healing approaches your own. I hope that they work as well for you as they have for me.

This series of entries describes how I learned to create emotionally healing experiences during my recovery from a rare childhood cancer and radical surgery. These experiences were not as bad as what some people face. But, perhaps they will encourage you to move through whatever difficulty you are facing now or help you to plan for the future. You can see how a young child learned on her own to employ memory and imagination to create visualizations of beloved green spaces and the creatures there. These were very effective in transporting me away from the trauma of surgery and hospital visits, helping me sleep, and helping me to gain some sense of control over body and mind. You can also see the great value of interactions with the natural world and its creatures, both wild and domesticated. I had a long way to go at that time, but things did continue to improve.

Age Four

The unmarred skin of my baby face brushes back and forth across the smooth, worn planks of the float, daring a tiny splinter to break free. My tongue slides across the salty board and into the space where that board nearly abuts the next one. Shards of golden light filter through the gaps between the planks. I push my face down hard against the wood, peering through a crack to see what lies beneath the water's surface. Hundreds of mussels cling by hairy threads to the corner posts, and clumps of seaweed gather up, providing shelter for the little fish that dart in and out. My nose scrunches up at the scent of gasoline mixed with the more appealing smells of the sea. What I'm really looking for appears out of the murk: a big old dogfish swims lazily toward a strip of light and moves back and forth beneath the float. I press my eye against the wood, trying to get a better view.

"Annie-pants, Annie-pants, ants in your pants, what'cha doin'?" I scramble to my feet to face the grinning "big boys." They are armed with fishing lines, and Cokes, and squished pink marshmallow-coated Twinkies. Johnnie shoves a grimy paw into his pocket and pulls out a Jawbreaker for me. "Sit down, little Annie-pants, and we'll show ya how ta fish. Bet yaw mommy doesn't know you're heah." He's right about that.

Cross-legged, I sit examining the jingle bells on my sneakers and the lace around the edges of my socks. The boys dangle their feet in the cold water and jerk their lines up and down methodically. "Got one," the brown-haired boy shouts. He has hair in his armpits, too. I can see it when he pulls on his line and hauls the wriggling dogfish out of the water. The dogfish thrashes on the dock, throwing water over us. Johnnie takes out his knife, bends down to the struggling fish, and slits its belly. Baby dogfish spill out of their mother, a wriggling mass of blood, and guts, and bodies.

The boys, hooting with glee and immersed in their activity, don't notice as I stand up and back toward the ramp. I feel hot and my stomach is sick as I run up the ramp, across the parking lot, and up the big hill toward my house. Slowing, I stick my hand up under my shirt to feel the scar that runs from the middle of my back all the way around to my tummy. It sticks up like a snake's body, mean and hard. I know the doctors cut me open to take something out. Did I have dogfish babies inside me, too?

I look back down the street toward the hill that goes down to the dock. There are probably lots of dogfish there now, and I hope the big boys aren't catching them. I get all shivery when I think about those dogfish babies. Oh, goodie, here come Bobby and Nat and Martha down Harraseeket. We all run into Brown's Market and head straight for the root beer popsicles. Running feels so good, and makes the bad feelings go away. So do my popsicle and my friends. Here come Sherry and Karen, too.

Karen's house is on one side of mine. Mr. Mayo and his parents, Mr. and Mrs. Toothacher, live on the other side. The Toothachers look like Santa and Mrs. Claus and are just as nice. Almost every day I visit them and have cookies and milk or hot chocolate. Sometimes we watch TV, sitting in their big stuffed chairs with trays in our laps. I'm not sure about Mr. Mayo. He is always in the garage sawing things. I try to make friends with him, but he doesn't have much to say. The most interesting thing about him is that he has this calendar with naked ladies on it. They all have enormous tops that stick out a long way. Not like my mom or me. Once I said, "Slim," (that's what my dad calls him and I thought it might be better than Mr. Mayo for this question), "how come you have those ladies on the wall?" He made some weird noise that sounded like a pig instead of answering me. I just can't figure him out. My parents say he's odd and that I should only visit the Toothachers. But I like going to Slim Mayo's garage and looking at the naked ladies. When I'm a grown-up lady, I would like to look like that blond one who has no marks or scars and has a great big top. If I had a top like that, I might go without a shirt, too. But, if I don't change, I will always wear a shirt because I don't want people to see me. Sometimes Karen, Bobby, Sherry, Martha, and Nat all go without shirts. But I don't because I am embarrassed. I wish I could tell someone, but I have to keep it secret. We don't talk about my scars or my operation because they are yucky.

Age Four and a Half

Miss Jones and Mrs. Jones live part way up Harraseeket. Miss Jones is a lady, but she doesn't have a husband. She is Mrs. Jones' daughter, and her father, Mr. Jones, died quite a long time ago. I think five years. Mrs. Jones is really old. Once she told me sixty.

That is a lot of years. Mrs. Jones and Miss Jones love it when I come to visit. I am not a bother, and they told me so.

Miss Jones and Mrs. Jones told me that they both had operations, too, and that they didn't die so I don't have to worry about getting to be five. That makes me feel better. Mr. Jones did die, though. They said he didn't have an operation when I asked them. He just died of a heart attack. I still am not sure that you don't die of operations, even though they said so. I will just have to wait and pray for each next birthday.

Age Five

We can't go swimming today because we have to go to Boston for my check-up. I hate going there because I always get carsick a lot, and when we get there, we don't have very much time in Boston Common—just time enough to get a big pink cotton candy and maybe a monkey on a stick. This time there are no stick monkeys in Boston Common so I choose a white Wowie cat to go with my old Wowie. Wowies are the softest thing and I need one in order to go to sleep. Their fur is not real cat fur. It is even softer. I don't think anyone would kill a cat to make a Wowie, but once I had a stuffed mouse that might have been real mouse fur. I carry my Wowie to the place where we park to go to the hospital.

Boston Children's Hospital is tall with lots of windows for all the sick children to look out. I don't think they get to see much because there are only more buildings—probably hospitals—that look the same. Gray and mean and scary. At least I don't have to stay in Children's Hospital anymore. But I did for a long time after my operation. Mommy and Daddy didn't tell me that. I just know it. I also know that the doctors took something awful out of me, and left me with lots of marks and scars that will never let me forget that I almost died. I hope I get to be six. Every night I pray, "Please, God, let me get to be six."

When I was four, every night when I said, "Now I lay me down to sleep," I kept praying "Please, God, let me get to be five," so I guess it worked. I will never stop praying to get to the next birthday. And the next Christmas. Right now I keep praying, "Please, God, let me get to be six," as we ride the elevator up to where I will see the doctor. He is famous, but I don't like him anyway. Mommy tells me I need to act nice, but I don't feel like it. I hate it when the doctors all look at me and make me be naked. I don't like their machines, and I don't think they keep me healthy. I think God does that because I pray and love him. He fixed me, not these doctors. And I hate Dr. Good, which is a stupid name for him because he always hurts me and gives me shots even though he does have lollypops and I can have as many as I want. But I only take one because I don't want him to think I like him even a little bit, but I do sort of like big fat Mrs. Skillin, his nurse. I choose root beer every time. Well, once I got cherry. So, when my Daddy was in law school and Mommy was home with me and wasn't a model or a newspaper person anymore, I got sick and Dr. Good found out and then I went to Children's Hospital for my operation and I almost lived there forever, I think. I hate the way my scars look and the other stuff, too, and I don't want anybody to look at me. I want my face to be beautiful like Mommy's so I can be a model, too, but I almost hate the rest of me. Well, not my arms and legs. They are good.

Mommy tells me I am beautiful. I even got first runner-up in the beautiful baby contest. Some Cheryl girl with more curls got first. I saw her in the newspaper. She probably doesn't have any scars and marks. But I did, even then, because I already had my operation. It is really important to be beautiful. Maybe even the most important thing. Just don't take off your clothes and they won't know.

These doctors in the hospital are stupid just like Dr. Good. There are too many of them, and they all look at me. Even if they try to be nice, I just want to go back to Sebago and go swimming. While we wait and wait for them and while they look at me, I just think about swimming, and I forget I am even at the hospital.

I love to dive off the big rock into the deep black water. The water is often cold, but it feels so clean and good on my skin when I am under the water with my hair streaming out behind me. I feel like I could just swim and swim with the minnows and the bass without ever coming up again. I can open my eyes under the water and see the schools of minnows and sometimes a bass or a spiny perch. Grand Daddy taught me about the kinds of fish. He and Uncle Ken and Daddy always take me fishing. I love fish and I don't want them to die, but I pretend I am happy when I catch them so no one else will feel bad. Before we cook them, Daddy traces the ones I catch and hangs the picture on the wall, right next to where I get measured and we mark it every time with the date and my age. That's fun, but I love live fish the most and swimming with them across the sandy bottom out to the really deep part where there are stones instead of sand. Maybe a snapping turtle lives there. Sometimes I think about them biting my toes when I can't see bottom, but I am not really worried. I love the turtles and all of the creatures (except spiders) because they make me happy and help to keep me from worrying about not getting to be the next age.

Everyone says I swim just like a fish. So why do we catch them and cut them down their bellies just like the doctors cut me? But I didn't die yet. Now I am crying and I just want to go back to Sebago, but I am right here in this hospital on this table and they made it so I couldn't even think about the swimming and the fish anymore.

Finally it's over, and they give me a balloon and some jellybeans and tell me I am a very good girl. I know they really are trying to be nice, and I pretend I like them. Even though I think all these bad things about them, I act polite, and I smile now and look pretty in my face like Mommy wants me to. I wish I could look pretty all over.

So, we walk back to the car and drive back to camp and I throw up some more, and then I just go to sleep. When we get back it is time for supper, but we get to go swimming off the big rock and I do some good dives. I do not want to go to Boston again for the hospital, but they told me I have to come until I am twelve years old. That is too much years for me to even think about, so instead of thinking about that when I go to bed, I think about Beddy Bear and swimming and about riding horses, too.

I have a baby sister, LoLo. I love her but she does not play with me and she does not go to the doctor's with me. She just gets the fun part. I still have to play with my bug friends by myself. I also have my friends that live down the register in the front hall. Mommy says they are imaginary, but they are not. They told me so.

Age Six

Running down the path from Nanny's camp to ours is one of my most favorite things. I love the way my feet fly across the ground, touching well-worn dirt in some places and padded-down grass in others. There are no roots or rocks that stick up—just the one smooth, flat rock that sits in the middle of the path halfway down the hill. Sometimes I stop and sit next to it, examining the little bluets that spring up around its edges. Their delicate blossoms grow in clusters and are easy to dig up and plant in a bowl. Nanny taught me that. She teaches me so many things. Like how to do the J-stroke, if I am canoeing from the stern, or how to work on the potters' wheel, or the difference between porcelain slip and regular slip when you're pouring a mold, or how to tell the difference between a red pine and a white pine, or an evening grosbeak from a rose-breasted grosbeak. Nanny is the best person in the world. She is an artist. Her sculptures of people like Admiral MacMillan are in museums. Her paintings and her hooked rugs are in lots of shows. I get to go to the art shows with her and to her painting group when it meets at Mere Point or at Miss Messenger's big yellow farmhouse. I think Miss Messenger's favorite people are ladies. All the artist ladies go there. Miss Messenger has flower gardens everywhere. She and Nanny tell me about delphiniums and peonies and about the difference between fairy roses and tea roses. I love learning about the flowers and studying their details and painting them with Nanny. When I get nervous, sometimes I just think about the roses, and I can almost smell their scent. Before I know it, all the beauty and everything that I am thinking about the flowers just takes me away, even if I can't really be in the garden right then.

Miss Messenger and Nanny both have antique doll collections. They let me change their pantaloons and dresses. I fix little tea parties for them, use the antique doll furniture, and carefully brush their hair and style it. They have real hair. Nanny even made a Diana doll that looks like me. She is not an antique. Nanny sculpted her head and made a wig of my hair after I had it cut. Her body is soft. She wears a blue hand-smocked dress just like mine, and she is three feet tall. My Diana doll doesn't have any marks or scars so I guess she didn't have an operation.

Age Seven

During so many nights, I wake up with dreams of spiders. I love all other living things, but spiders terrify me. In my dream, I am in a metal crib with bars all around. There is a window near my bed that allows the sunlight to flow into the room. I like watching the way the shadows dance upon the walls. The scary part of my dream comes when a huge gray spider peers up over the edge of my blanket and begins to move slowly toward me. It meanders across my covers, coming closer and closer. In a panic, I struggle to get away but my hands and feet are tied and the spider comes closer. Soon it has reached my neck. I scream and scream, but no one comes. The spider walks across my face and head and disappears somewhere behind my curls. I scream and thrash so much that the ties on my wrists and ankles cut through my tender skin again. The nurse I love most of all comes into my room, bandages my sore spots, strokes my head, and sings to me. I'm not scared any more, but my wrists and ankles hurt.

When I wake up from the dream, I turn on my light to be sure there are no spiders in my bed. I touch the soft skin on my wrists and ankles, tracing the thin raised lines that mar them. In all, I have five scars: these four and my enormous one. I stay at Nanny's camp now with her because a spider got on me once in the night when I was in my bunk bed at our camp. I won't sleep there now because it is scary. I wish I could remember why I hate spiders, but I can't even though I keep trying. I think it has something to do with my scars.

Age Nine

My birthday this year is going to be the best ever. Mom is making me a Cinderella cake with a pumpkin coach that will be drawn by eight ceramic horses. I love all horses. Just thinking about them makes me happy. We are having the party in our barn, and I am inviting everyone in my class, plus some of the older kids, too. Mom is weaving a huge string spider's web in one dark corner. That is kind of weird because I hate spiders; fortunately, it will not be full of live spiders. Mom is vacuuming the barn to get rid of the live ones. I feel guilty about killing them, but I am so scared. I wish I wasn't such a baby. Anyway, each person will get a very long string that winds its way through the web. At the end of our string we will each find a special present that is wrapped in black or orange tissue paper. I wanted everyone to have a present at my party because some of my friends have never even had a birthday party. You know, parties are just the best thing because they make everyone happy. I love seeing all of my friends having fun, plus when we have parties I don't even think about dying. That is a pretty good thing considering how much time I spend worrying about it. Sometimes when I am worried, I plan parties in my head right down to every little detail like what the decorations will look like on the cake. I like to plan the cakes with real roses that smell so great scattered all over them. Over and over I go, planning lots of parties in my head so that I will stay happy. Maybe if I ever get to be grown up, I will be a party girl.

I love my new school, my teacher, all of my new friends, and our house. It is all fixed up and beautiful compared to what it was when we bought it. On the outside it was really pretty, but the inside was a mess. Now our house is beautiful and has a new kitchen, too, which Mom really likes. I want to be like our house, with a cleaned up body from my neck to my legs. No scars. Maybe Mom would think I looked beautiful enough.

One place we have to go soon again is for my appointment at Boston Children's Hospital, but I don't want to think about that now. I just had Dr. Good, my pediatrician, at the end of the summer, and that was bad enough. When Dr. Good gave me my shot, the needle broke off in my arm and I was screaming. Mrs. Skillin had to come in, and hold me down while he pulled out the needle, and then he said he had to give me another shot. So I jumped off the table and ran out the door and down the hall into another room. I slammed the door, but it had no lock so I crawled under the desk to hide. Mom, Mrs. Skillin, and Dr. Good all came in and tried to get me out, but I wasn't about to go back for another shot. I figured I would just stay there until dark and wait for them to leave. Then I would figure out how to find Mom and Daddy and our car so I could go home and never come back to Dr. Good. But my plan didn't work because enormous Mrs. Skillin, who is also really strong, got down on her stomach on the floor and kept grabbing toward me. I couldn't squish back any further, so she caught me and started pulling me out from under the desk. She had to really pull hard, which hurt my leg enough so that it had a red mark for two days, probably because on the way out I grabbed one of the legs of the desk and held on. Before she caught me, I could see that her face was all red and puffy and that she had hairs sticking out of her nose. Mrs. Skillin is what my dad would call "unattractive," but she is probably nice to her grandchildren. She is actually nice to me, too, but Mom said she was probably "fed up" with me. It wasn't her arm that the needle was in. Or Mom's. By the way, Dr. Good did give me another shot while I was on the floor. I am fed up with all of them and their shots.

I was about to tell what happened on the second day of school. I was trying to remember all the kids' names, and how to get home from school in case Sue was ever sick, and all the other stuff you need to know when you are new. Sometimes it is so hard for me to go in the right direction. Uncle Ken says I couldn't find my way out of a paper bag. Anyway, at recess, we were all swinging and having a really great time with the big kids giving us dunks. That's when you push the swing way up in the air and run under it so the person in the swing gets a great ride. It is really fun to get dunks. The only problem was that, after my turn, Rodney was trying to show me how to give dunks even though I'm not tall enough. Rodney is in sixth grade and very tall and skinny, with nice crinkly eyes and a big toothy smile. Anyway, he gave this really big push and Danny fell out of the swing when Rodney dunked him. Danny was sort of okay, except he needed some iodine and two bandaids for his elbow, I guess. But the swing came back really fast without Danny in it and hit me in the head. I don't really remember, but all the kids said I fell right down on the ground and they thought I was dead. I am so scared of dying, but I didn't think it would happen from being hit in the head by a swing. The kids said Mrs. Carter, she's the principal and the fifth grade teacher in case you forgot, came running over, even though she is very fat and old and I can't imagine her running. In a minute, or maybe two, my eyes opened and the nurse came and I had to go to her office until they said it was okay to go back to my room. I kept crying for a long time, which was pretty bad because I cried the day before when I was worried about getting lost going home, too. I hoped no one would call me a crybaby, but only one kid did and no one likes him anyway.

Sometimes I think I cry too much. I cry when I get hurt, when I get scared, when I need to talk in front of people, when someone yells at me, when Daddy spanks me, and when I think about dying, which is a lot of time. I just can't help it. It comes up inside of me and makes me choke before the tears come. Sometimes I just cry without any tears but with all kinds of sadness. Sometimes I am happy though, like when I am riding Pom Pom or grooming him, or swimming with the fish, or running down the hill from Nanny's camp to ours.

Then at the end of the week we had to write a poem for homework so I wrote this one about seagulls:

Where do the gulls go at night?
I wonder as I watch them in their flight. They may go to the hills or into
the sky Or maybe to the cliffs they fly. Where do the gulls go at night?
I wonder as I watch them in their flight.

Everyone in my class loved my poem, especially the way I wrote it on my daddy's fancy paper and decorated it all around the edges with pictures of seagulls and hills and water scenes. I got an A + which made me so happy. I love A plusses, and so the week turned out really good after all.

Age Ten

Bad Dream

It is dark and I am alone. The thickly wooded trail winds on and on. I know that I need to reach the second field in order to find the path back to the safety of the Rivers' house, but each time I think I am nearly there, confusion and panic overwhelm me. Tears pour down my face, blurring my vision. I will never get home. I will die here in the woods, the animals will pick my bones clean, and in a hundred years a little boy will dig through the leaves looking for salamanders and instead will find my skull.

Another Bad Dream

I am in the attic of our house. I love going there because I can feel all the people who lived in this beautiful place with its elegant rooms and circular staircase. Mom and Dad say they have given this house back its soul and restored it to its former dignity. All the people who lived here are grateful. I hear their ghosts sighing in the night, the weight of their footsteps padding up the stairs to the third floor to the attic room where our leather-bound trunk of antique clothes rests, awaiting their approval. The fragile lacy wedding gown fits my thin body almost perfectly and reminds me of how small my ancestors must have been. The people of this house must have been tiny, too. Mrs. Carver, whose manicured hand glided lovingly over the banister, her button shoes tapping on the stairs as she wound her way up, up through the third floor to the cupola, where she would anxiously await the first glimpse of her husband as his ship's sails approached the harbor after months at sea. Stern-faced Captain Carver, who presided over this place even when he was thousands of miles away in the Orient loading his ship. Their strawberry blonde daughter in her dotted-swiss dress, leading her yellow tabby cat by a brown leather leash, who now gazes out from the portrait that hangs next to her parents' in our dining room. These inhabitants came with the house. Years later we learn that the Carvers are closely related to my grandmother and that Captain Carver's ship likely sailed the same routes as our family vessels, plying the trade with the Orient.

The Carvers are with me in the attic until I spot the tiny doorway at the back. Then they vanish, and I am alone, knowing that I must unlock the door and squeeze through into the dark passageway beyond. I enter and crawl along the passageway, feeling the rough-hewn wood and pegged corners, anticipating all that lies ahead. Suddenly, the awareness that huge furry black spiders also inhabit this tunnel fills me with panic. I try to turn around, but have no room to maneuver. I crawl backward, splinters stabbing my hands and knees, as I realize the passage is growing smaller. Thankfully, my feet reach the open door, only to discover that the rest of my body will not fit through. I am stuck with the spiders that have now crawled over my face and neck. I kick and scream. There is a great crash and the sound of shattering glass.

Awake

I am awake, soaked in sweat with tears flowing from my eyes, in my comfy cannonball bed, the house silent, my fish tanks bubbling away. It is Christmas morning. In the early dawn glow, I creep down the stairs hoping to beat the rest of the family to the tree. As I round the corner to the living room, I discover the tree lying on the floor surrounded by shards of blue, green, silver, and gold. Gray Baby lies comfortably in the midst of it all. He stirs and watches me with one sleepy cat eye, stretches, and ambles over for some hugs. Gray Baby is a big, rugged Russian Blue—a far cry from the scrawny, wet kitten I hauled out of a paper bag in the Mount Ephraim Brook last September. Mom cautioned me that his chances for survival were slim, but he proved everyone wrong. Sort of like me, I guess.

Even though I have bad dreams at night, almost every day here is so much fun. My new friends all had such a great time at my Halloween birthday party in the barn, plus they came to our house for a big Christmas party, too. Our house is a perfect party house, Mom says. Maybe I can have another Halloween birthday if I get to be eleven. Plus we have our own frog pond that is also great for skating. In the fall I brought newts and frogs from the pond to live in some of my tanks for the winter. My favorite newt, Sir Isaac, climbed out of his tank and was missing for 10 days. Mom said he probably dried up under my bed, but I kept praying that he would come home to his tank. With a little help, he did! One day when we were at school Mom found him walking right down the hall toward one of my doors. He was all covered with dust balls and had a big trail of dust that he was pulling along behind him, which means that he probably was under a bed. But, he was not dried up! I am so happy to have Sir Isaac back again. God saved Sir Isaac Newt and maybe he can save me, too. I am so happy here in our beautiful house, with all of my pets, in a new town where no one knows about my operation or my ugly body. We are far away from Boston Children's Hospital.

Tomorrow when we go to school, we have a man coming to visit our room who will be making identification charts for us. If we are ever lost, this will help people find us. We are all excited to have our charts made, plus we might even get to have our fingerprints taken. The only thing I am not happy about now is that we have to go to Children's Hospital soon for my appointment. I wish LoLo could go instead of me, but she didn't have an operation so all she has to do is have fun in Boston. My whole family likes going to Boston except me. I wish I could stay here with Sue. LoLo wishes she could have had an operation so she would get more special presents when we go to Children's Hospital. She can have the ones the doctors give me.

No Fun

So, the man from the FBI came to our class today. Instead of being fun it ended up being one of the worst days of my life. We were all sitting in our seats listening to him talk about protecting children from being lost, which was really interesting. Plus he told us he brought his fingerprinting equipment. Every person has different fingerprints that can be used for identification. Sometime the FBI would like to have fingerprints of all the children in the country so every lost child could be found. I hope that happens because I was lost once and it was terrifying at first. Mommy and I were walking along the street holding hands, and I kept trying to let go, so finally she let me walk next to her. Everything went fine for a while, and then she just wasn't there. I was only four, so I cried and cried until someone found me and took me in a store because my mother had lost me. Then they put a chair in the window of the store, between all of the towels and sheets, and told me to sit in the chair so my mom would see me when she walked by. They gave me some tootsie rolls, which made me a little bit happier, but I was still worrying quite a lot. Finally, Mommy came and knocked on the window at me. After she thanked all the people in the store, we went to the drug store and got an ice cream before we met Daddy and drove home. Even though it turned out fine for me, I hope no other children get lost. If they do, I hope the FBI can find them if their mothers can't.

Even though the FBI man was trying to help all of us today, it ended up bad for me. When we were doing our charts, Mrs. Light kept going around the class asking the same question for each of us while the FBI man wrote down the answers. Most of the questions were okay. They were just about who we were, who our parents were, and where we lived. Then the awful question came.

"Do you have any identifying marks or scars?" asked Mrs. Light. Everyone was saying things like, "How big does it have to be?" "If I cut my finger once and had stitches, does that count?" "I have a mole on my arm." They were all excited about having some kind of little mark that could go on their chart to help to identify them.

I was frozen in my seat and felt like I was going to throw up. By the time Mrs. Light got to Danny's seat, which is two seats in front of mine, I wanted to get up and run out of the room. Danny said he had a scar where he broke his arm. Mrs. Light asked how long it was. When Danny told her two inches, everyone said, "EEOOU, that's disgusting." I decided right then I was not telling about my scar. If everyone thought Danny's two inch scar was disgusting what would they think when I said I had a big thick scar that went almost all the way around me? Probably no one would even like me any more.

Then Mrs. Light got to Ruthie who said she had no marks or scars, but she did have a little teeny mole on her cheek, so Mrs. Light told the man to put that down. I could feel my face getting really hot and I just knew I was going to cry if I had to talk. I had already decided not to tell about my scar, which made me into a liar, so I knew I had to say something about my mark. "Diana, do you have any identifying scars?"

"No," I said while I looked down at my desk and tried not to cry.

"What about any identifying marks?"

I kept my head looking down so no one would see the tears and answered, "Yes," very softly.

"Please speak up, Diana, we couldn't hear you. Do you have any identifying marks?"

I just knew everyone in the whole class was looking at me. I answered "Yes" louder. Then Mrs. Light asked me how big my mark was so I lied again and said, "Not too big."

"About the size of a dime?" asked Mrs. Light.

"Bigger," I mumbled.

"You have to speak up, Diana, so we can properly record your answers. Now, how big is your mark? Is it the size of a quarter or a half dollar?"

Then I told another huge lie when I answered, "A quarter." My mark is really as big as half my whole body. By now I was shaking and could see the tears making a puddle on my desk.

"What color is your mark, Diana?"

"Brown."

"Where is your mark, Diana?"

Well, that was a problem, because I didn't know which part to choose, my stomach, my back or my arm. I also was not going to say one thing about the scar. I took so long answering that Mrs. Light sounded very impatient when she said, "You really need to give your answers so the whole class can have their turn, Diana. Now where is your mark?"

"Under my arm," I lied again.

"Under arm perspiration," Danny whispered so loud that every-one in the whole class could hear him. Most of the boys, plus Bonnie, laughed, and Mrs. Light put their names on the board.

"Linda, how about you? Do you have any identifying scars or marks?"

"I have a little purple birthmark behind my right ear," Linda replied proudly. "My mom says it makes me special." I just sat in my chair, trying to be as small as possible by shrinking way down in my seat. I didn't feel very special. I felt like a freak. Maybe if I get to be twelve the doctors can erase my marks and make me normal before I get to be through with Children's Hospital. If I get to be twelve, I don't have to go there ever again. And, if I ever get to be twelve, I am changing my name to Dianna, instead of Diana, because I want to be new.

Lying

I am spending quite a lot of time worrying about my lying to Mrs. Light and the FBI man. I know liars don't go to heaven, so what happens if I die before I am eleven?

It is important not to get into the worrying because then the nightmares come every night. The wolf nightmares are the worst ones because the wolves keep chasing me trying to kill me. Sometimes my legs won't move the right way, and no matter how much I try, I can't get away from the wolves. When my legs won't run in the dream, it is like being stuck in deep clay or, I guess, quicksand, even though I don't really know what quicksand is like. I can only imagine it because of how they describe it on the Roy Rogers show. The bad guys always get stuck in quicksand. I know I am not as bad as the outlaws on Roy Rogers, but I did lie to Mrs. Light and the FBI man. The wolf nightmares started way before that though. Every night when I say my prayers, I say a silent prayer about getting to be the next year older instead of dying and about not having the wolf nightmares. Mostly, the nightmare prayer doesn't work, but I am just glad the "next birthday prayer" is working. At least so far.

God told me to think good things instead of bad things and to stop the worrying. I am trying to do that. I think about all my friends and my pets, our pretty house, my family, camp, and horses. I am going to work on thinking more about horses when I am having trouble sleeping and feeling scared of dying or of wolves eating me. Beddy Bear used to work for me when I thought about him, but now I guess I need to think more about horses because Beddy Bear seems like he is more for little kids, like Wowie was for babies.

Beddy Bear is my fluffy white bear who I used to pretend was talking to me and helping me go to sleep. He said all sorts of kind things to me and told me how to get all comfy in my bed. He kept telling me I wouldn't die. After listening to him for a while, I would just go to sleep.

It is really a relief to have gotten to be ten. Things are getting better. The "horse thoughts" have been keeping the wolf dreams and the worrying about dying away. Every night after my prayers I think really hard about horses. The first thing I do is close my eyes and get a picture in my mind of Pom Pom. It's almost like looking at television because I can see everything about him. *He is quite a chubby horse and only 14.2 hands tall. Within his shape, I see the clearly defined brown and white patches on his coat that make him a piebald. I can see his stiff black mane and tail that are sometimes hard to comb through. I imagine brushing his coat and watching it turn sleek and shiny. I inhale his wonderful horse smell. Then I watch myself tacking him up and leading him out of his stall into the stable yard. I put his reins over his head and take them in my left hand while putting my hand on his withers. I stretch my left leg up, put it in the stirrup, and swing myself into the saddle. I urge Pom Pom forward with some slight pressure, and we trot out of the stable yard up toward the ring. We trot out around the ring, do a few figure-eights, and go back to the rail. I collect him down by sitting deep into my saddle and flexing my reins slightly. Then I give him the canter signal, and he moves forward into his choppy little canter. In my horse thoughts, I give Pom Pom a long, graceful stride and a smooth canter. That is a much more comfortable stride for me, and I might as well give it to him since I can change anything I want when I am in my horse thoughts.*

Sometimes I have already fallen asleep by the time Pom Pom is back out on the rail for the canter. If I haven't, I just keep going with my horse images. The more I focus on the images, the less I think about anything around me that is not a part of the horse thoughts. The worrying always goes away, and when I come out of the horse thoughts (or, if I am going to sleep for the night, when I wake up the next morning) I am feeling relaxed and happy. No wolves or dying worries have been able to get into my mind because my mind is so full of horse thoughts that there is no room for them. If I fall down and cut myself in real life, I can go into horse thoughts and not even feel the pain.

I have my "galloping free horse thoughts" that I like to think about sometimes, too. Then I am riding Blaze Away, the tall black thoroughbred with the white blaze down his face, who Nanny painted a picture of me riding.

We are at the top of Canter Hill in Nanny's painting, but in my horse thoughts we begin at the bottom of Canter Hill and gallop up through the tall grasses. The fields stretch ahead as far as I can see, and we continue to gallop effortlessly through them. I can feel the late summer breeze soft against my face as we go on and on. Ahead I see a stone wall and focus on it as I urge Blaze Away forward. I prepare for the jump, and Blaze Away pricks his ears ahead, eager for the jump, and makes a sound, muscular departure from the field into the air. We fly over the jump and feel complete freedom as we glide through the air, return to the ground, and gallop on toward an endless series of fields and jumps. We gallop on and on for as long as I want. In my mind, I am only on Blaze Away, soaring over the jumps and galloping easily across the fields. Nothing else is in my mind at all. When I go to Children's Hospital next week, I am going to go into "galloping-free horse thoughts" the whole time I am there.

Because there are some other things I like in addition to horses, I focus on them sometimes, too. Once when I wanted to get out of worrying and go to sleep, I imagined *getting into our canoe with Nanny and canoeing across smooth waters just before sunset way out onto Sebago Lake. I could see and feel each stroke of my paddle as it sliced through the water and came up sprinkling little silver drops from its blade as I feathered to stroke again. While the sun dropped lower in the sky behind the purple hills that sit in front of Mount Washington, I watched the colors begin to deepen. With the last glimpse of the sun, the sky filled with red, orange, purple, and violet. The streaks of color stretched out across the sky, reflecting in the now-darkening waters of the lake. Then I saw the colors gradually begin to fade away as the sky began to go to black and get ready to welcome the stars.* When I woke up the next morning, I felt peaceful and relaxed. I found myself thinking about Sebago and how much I love it there.

Last summer I began using my mind to help me to do better in my swimming and diving. When I wasn't even in the water, I would imagine that I was preparing for a dive. I would remember all the things that I knew about diving and sometimes put myself in the body of someone who I knew was an excellent diver. In my mind I would rehearse the dive over and over until it seemed like the most natural thing in the world to do that perfect dive. Then, when I did the dive in real life, it was easier and better than ever. I think that practicing with my imagination will help me do better at everything.

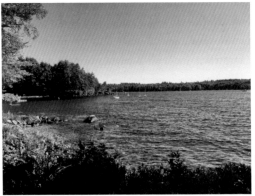

Healing Waters of Sebago Lake.

DIARIES AND MEMORIES: PART II

A GRIEVING ADOLESCENT MOVES ON
TO A HEALTHIER PLACE

"The very winds whispered in soothing accents,
and maternal Nature bade me weep no more."
Mary Shelley

While I have some hesitation about sharing more of my own life experiences, I am going to do it anyway. Regardless of what you are facing now or what the future holds, so many of us have been there as well. Whether we are encountering the effects of aging, dealing with the regular ups and downs of life, feeling overwhelmed by responsibility, or coping with some medical crisis, we can find solace in knowing that someone else has been there. As you think through your own issues, I hope this diary from my youth will help you to approach your challenges in a constructive manner. My tales represent an unedited childhood diary where alternative healing approaches and green space engagement made the difference between just getting by and having a good life.

Age Eleven

Today we have the Synchers synchronized swimming show. We have practiced all summer and are really good so I don't want to mess anything up. I am really nervous about doing everything perfectly, but most of all I am nervous about my bathing suit. I have a better chance of being a perfect Syncher than I do of looking perfect in this bathing suit. We voted on bathing suits last week. Everyone except me wanted to wear the two-piece checked ones like so many of the seniors have. They come in blue, pink, or yellow and white checks and are really cute. I used to wish I had one, but I wouldn't wear it if I did, so what's the point? Now I have to wear the one I borrowed from Caroline so that all the Synchers will be dressed the same. I couldn't be the only one who voted against these suits, so I pretended I thought it was a great idea and voted for them. Now I am about to die of embarrassment. You can probably figure out the problem. We have to walk all the way down the stone pier past all the guests who are coming to the show and then out onto the metal pier, where we will dive in to begin our routine. Somehow I have to make it past about a hundred guests plus 106 campers and counselors without them seeing all my marks and scars, which is probably impossible. I don't want to wreck the Synchers show by looking awful in this bathing suit, but I probably will. I will just have to put my brain in another place while I am walking down that pier. When I went to Dr. Bad before camp started, I tried to be really brave and ask him about sandpaper surgery, a technique I read about in a magazine. It said you can get rid of scars and birthmarks by sanding them away. I could tell my mother was humiliated when I asked Dr. Bad this question, probably because she wishes she had a daughter who was perfect and she got stuck with *me*. I will always have to leave everything out between my neck and my legs. Dr. Bad laughed at me and asked why I would want to have sandpaper surgery, which was about the stupidest question in the world, and I said, "So I can wear a two-piece bathing suit, (Stupid)."

(I only thought the "Stupid" part.) He just kept laughing stupidly and said, "Diana, you will look beautiful in a two-piece bathing suit just the way you are. No one will be able to take their eyes off you." Which is what I am afraid of right now. So, that was the end of the sandpaper surgery idea. After about a year of planning how I would ask him about it, he just laughed me off, and my mother just stood there smiling. So now here I am standing here with my towel wound around me, pretending that I am cold when it's about 90 degrees, dreading the minute when the music starts and I have to drop my towel and parade down the pier with the rest of the Synchers. I hate my mother and Dr. Bad for not giving me sandpaper surgery. (By now you have probably figured out that I have renamed Dr. Good "Dr. Bad.")

Oh, my God, the music is starting and there goes my towel. I start smiling and walking in this weird way with my body kind of twisted around and my arms slightly twisted, too, trying to turn my body away so it won't show, and cranking my head around to look at the audience, and still do what I'm supposed to do in the entrance walk. That normally wouldn't be hard for me at all since it's like ballet and I've had plenty of that. If only I had on a regular bathing suit. Then I would only have to twist my right arm in, which I am used to doing any time I have on a bathing suit or anything sleeveless. If I'd had sandpaper surgery, there would be no problem, and maybe I could have a normal life.

I have almost made it down the pier with all this twisting, but I'm sure that at least Syd and Lillian saw me. They are our camp directors. Now I'm worrying about what I am going to do when I get out of the water and have to parade all the way back down both piers facing the crowd. Thank God, I have made it to the line-up on the metal pier. We dive in one at a time and, when my turn comes, I know I've made a perfect dive as my body slips through the cool water and I surface in position. I love synchronized swimming even better than racing, even though I'm good at that, too. My mind just drifts away from all of the things I hate and am scared of. It is much better than ballet where I am always blind because I won't wear those stupid glasses. Everything is closer in the water. The whole show is going perfectly, and we all look like little seals. Everyone is clapping with enthusiasm, so I know they love our routine and think we are all doing a great job, which we are. Here comes the grand finale, and once again it goes just right. We are all swimming toward the ladder and climbing out to do our exit walk. Here I go again. Hopefully, I am dripping enough that the water will cover me up as much as a towel, but probably not. I've almost made it back to where Caroline is holding my towel. When I get there, she says, "That's a really cool scar you have. Why didn't you show me that before? I love scars." God, she is so weird sometimes, but this is the weirdest. I wish she would just shut up before someone else hears her and starts asking about scars. Next year I am not wearing a two-piece bathing suit for the show if I get to be on Synchers again, which I think I will because in my heart I know I am one of the best. By the way, now that summer is going by, soon it will be October and you know what that means. I will be twelve! Done forever with Boston Children's Hospital! I can also be Dianna, instead of Diana. I am going to be new!

Age Sixteen

This is going to be the most amazing year of my life. I am finally going to be a senior! I have had a fun summer doing horses and being out-doors. I love Sebago Lake and camp. In lots of ways I feel like the luckiest person I know—even though I wouldn't say that to anybody. To tell the truth, I never thought I'd get to be this old. All those birth-days, since I was just a tiny little kid, I prayed that I would get to have another birthday the next year. I prayed to have another Christmas, to have a horse, to earn my Curved Bar, to make cheering every year, to win on the swim team and in the broad jump, to be on Synchers, to get my Advanced in stuff at camp, to be a good friend, and to not get sick again. Sometimes I just can't believe it's all going the way I hoped. There have been times when I didn't think it was going to happen this way at all. Now I am having fun with Jill and our new friends from Gray and North Windham. Jill is my best friend ever, and she makes everything so much fun. I can tell her almost anything. She is funny, pretty, sensitive, smart, and an excellent writer. I wish I could write as well as she does. We even go on double dates. My boyfriends have gone back to college, but I think I am getting another one. This year is going to be great.

Last year, I thought everything was going better. Then I started waking up in the morning feeling really bad. I would just lie there trying to decide how bad the feeling was—whether it was going to be a bad day or a good day. Some days everything seemed absolutely black, and I couldn't even think about going to school. There never seemed to be any reason for it. I just had this sense of impending doom. To avoid going to school, I would put hot water in my mouth before Mom took my temperature. I guess she didn't really notice that I didn't go to school the day after games for almost the whole season. Nobody at school had a clue either, except maybe Jill. I was worrying all the time. Even though I was Varsity Cheering Captain, on the swim team, on a ton of other things, and had a great boyfriend, nothing really felt right. I didn't tell anybody else this, but I spent a lot of time thinking about dying and how I probably would never get to be a senior, go to college, go to grad school, get married, or have a baby. It just seemed like I had lucked out for too many years.

I still don't know what was wrong with me when I was a baby, but I guess it must have been pretty bad or they wouldn't have cut me absolutely in half when they did my operation. You just wouldn't do that to a little baby unless you thought there was no other way to give them a chance to live. So I really did luck out, I guess, in so many ways.

There were a few years when I really didn't want to be with either of my parents. I can remember being on trips and pretending I didn't even know them. I'd walk really fast, way out in front of them, and not answer when they called my name. As a matter of fact, when I was twelve and stopped going to Children's Hospital, I even changed my name from Diana to Dianna just to let them know that I was in charge. Also, changing my name could make me into a new person who could be more perfect. I am learning how to keep the secrets about my operation and my ugly body and how to use just my face for people.

You wouldn't believe some of the things those doctors did to me. The last time I went to Children's Hospital, when I was twelve, they examined me and did all their tests. Then they made me stand absolutely naked in front of everyone while a photographer took pictures of me. It was humiliating and probably damaged me for life. Maybe I should be a psychiatrist and treat all the children who have been messed up by doctors. Nobody has ever even told me what was wrong with me in all these years either. Every time I ask, I get some inane answer like, "Don't worry about it. You're fine now." Well, I do worry about it, and I also spend half my life worrying about dying. I tried to talk to our school counselor about my worries once, but he spent the whole time blushing, mumbling, and generally acting stupid. I can't talk to anyone else, because you really shouldn't complain or tell anyone else personal things. Oh well, so much for that. I am definitely better off than I was last year and the years before that.

Senior Year, Back in School

Christmas vacation is over, and we are back in school. Everything is the same yet nothing is the same. Dad has been in the hospital since the day after New Year's. He got to come home for one night and get his clothes, and I haven't seen him since then. I don't know what is wrong with him, and Mom won't tell me. I've been driving her to the hospital, but she doesn't want me to come in. Nanny is going to be taking her from now on so I can start going to my practices again. My new camera is just sitting there waiting for Dad. I guess he'll be home pretty soon, but it's already been six days. I feel so depressed and worried.

My life feels as if it has two distinct components that are incompatible. Each day I head off to school and play the perfect little teenager. I sit in classes and walk the corridors at break with a smile pinned to my face, never talking to anyone about what is really going on inside my head and heart. I fear that my obsession with having everything perfect may be very hard on the cheering squads. We practice to the point of exhaustion, look great when we do our routines at games, and get lots of compliments from the crowd. What is weird, though, is that I often feel confused about the cheers and have these panicky sensations before we go on the floor to perform—not such a great thing since I am the captain. My sleep is disrupted by nightmares about getting out in front of a huge crowd and not remembering what to do. I also dream about forgetting for weeks to feed my horse. Then I find him dead in the stall when I finally do remember he's out there in the barn.

In the mornings I am back into weighing my emotions like I did last year, evaluating whether it's going to be a decent day or a black day before I even get out of bed. It's as if my head just can't keep everything straight: all the things at school like play practice, cheering, swim team, yearbook, and classes; modeling assignments, my Teenaged Express newspaper work, and college applications; trying to spend as much time as possible with Doug while avoiding the drinking; my overwhelming worries about Dad and my irritation with Mom for, as usual, not talking about what is really going on. If only there was someone to talk to who could really understand my feelings. I don't even talk to my friends about things because I don't want to be boring. My time with Jill is when I just cut loose because she will put up with me no matter how I act.

It has been a month since I first took Dad to the doctor's and he was hospitalized.

Neither Lois nor I have seen him since then. Much of my free time has been spent on the college applications. I have put them in two categories: the ones that I picked myself and really want to go to and the ones that Mom and Dad picked for me. Theirs are not going to get much attention because I have my own ideas about what I want to do with my life. Mom thinks I should be an English major, but my plan is to be a psychiatrist and work with teenagers. I have mostly given up on the ideas of biology and surgery as careers because I think there is such a critical need for kids my age to have access to people who really understand their emotions and want to help them. They need to be able to talk to people who are well educated in their field, not just losers like my guidance counselor, who talks about my great potential while he looks me up and down. He never even asks about Dad.

Our play director wanted me to try out for the part of the young wife, but I refused. I only wanted to be the nine-year-old daughter who spends a lot of time roller-skating around the stage and acting silly. I got the part and like falling into that role at practice. Then I can just be the little kid with no worries, although in my real life I had plenty of worries about dying when I was little.

I keep trying to get notes to be excused from physical education, despite the fact that I love tumbling and using the trampoline. For the last few years I have been relatively successful at showering and changing off in a corner of the locker room so that no one could see my body, but now weird Miss Lane insists that she check us for water to be sure we are showering. I refuse to stand naked in front of her or anyone else. I had enough of that when I was being scrutinized at Children's Hospital for about eleven years. No one else is ever going to tell me when to take my clothes off again. She can flunk me for all I care. Once a week I can get away with not going to her class by pretending I am sick and staying home from school. On the other day, I either get a note from Mom saying I have a stomach ache or I forge one saying that I have the curse.

Dad at Home

Dad is home. He has been transformed from a round Dad with a rosy face into a shrunken old gray-complected man with cavernous eyes and sunken cheeks. He has all these bags hanging off him because he can't go to the bathroom, and that presents all kinds of unpleasant complications. I promise that when he's better I will be nicer and more loving when I am around him. I know he realizes that he smells and that he feels bad about it, but it is all I can do to even give him a quick kiss good night. He keeps telling me that when he is better, we will work on photography together and that next summer we'll do a lot of fishing. There are about three months between now and summer so there's plenty of time for him to get well even before my play and before graduation. I also have the senior prom and lots of swim meets before then. Dad says he wants to take a lot of pictures of all those things so I can have a great photo album of my senior year. Please let him get well soon.

Life

The days go by in a blur, while the nights stretch on forever. Just when I get to sleep, my clanging alarm clock sounds and I have to get ready for school. In order not to need more time in the morning and to be able to stay in bed a little longer, each night I put out my clothes for the next day. I have a chart of all of my outfits and plan ahead what I am going to wear. Tomorrow is my day for my hounds tooth skirt with the brown ribbed sweater. I have a headband that matches my skirt that I will also wear. I have charts for everything now so that I will know exactly what is coming next.

There is only one thing that I can't put on a chart and that is Dad and our future with him. Yesterday after school Lo, Mom, and I went to the hospital to visit him. Lo and I had never been inside before because Mom usually won't let us get out of the car.

It was a bleak, rainy March day, and the hospital loomed up from the sidewalk making no promise of anything positive. We rode the elevator up to Dad's floor and walked silently down the corridor. Nuns swept past us in their habits and spoke to Mom. I guess they all know her fairly well by now.

I could see a shape connected to all sorts of tubes when I started in the door of Dad's room. I soon realized that the unrecognizable form was my father. In the few short weeks since he was at home, he had lost so much more weight that he looked like a skeleton. Everything about him was gray, weak, and depressed. He had barely enough strength to speak to us and kept drifting off to sleep.

Why has Mom kept us away from him? It is clear to me that there is no hope of a recovery. It's too late to be able to have even a normal conversation. If only I had been told what was happening. Then I wouldn't have squandered my days and evenings focusing on my own life. Why couldn't Mom have let me go with her to the hospital each day, instead of having Nanny drive her or making me wait outside in the car?

When the nurse told us our visiting time was up, I walked numbly into that sterile corridor. The nuns seemed to be everywhere—black crows flapping in all directions with silly smiles on their faces. When we got in the elevator with some of them, I started yelling at Mom and Lo, "Don't you know he's going to die? He's already almost there!" I guess the nuns tried to calm me down, and I just went silent. I have nothing to say to anyone now. I will not see my father again. I know it. Yet I have to go to school and practices and do all of the other normal life things without showing anyone that I am only a shell. Just like my dad. Even though no one has ever said the word, I know he has cancer. And I know cancer kills almost everyone it touches. Did I have cancer, too?

Unraveling

I can't keep track of anything. I keep forgetting what time I have scheduled practices and where I have put my stuff. Yesterday I got to school and realized I had left my book bag home with all my assignments in it. And, I forgot to write down that we have a quiz today in French IV. I think I am going insane or something. It's lucky that I already got into some colleges. They probably wouldn't want some insane person. Remember, I told you that I divided my colleges into the ones my parents wanted and the ones I wanted? I never sent the applications in to some of the ones my parents chose, and on the rest I only filled in some of the answers. I didn't get into any of them except for two, thankfully. But, I got into all of my choices. I did not tell Mom this because she has too much to worry about with Dad, and she will be upset that I put in serious applications only to girls' colleges. Of course, she doesn't know that I applied to them anyway. That will be a big surprise for her when I make my choice. She thinks it is really important to go to school with guys and have dates every Friday and Saturday night.

Dad is still in the hospital. I don't know when he is coming home again, and I feel really guilty about the way I acted when he was here. Maybe they will take all of those tubes out of him soon and he will start to get better. I don't know.

Every night I have nightmares about Dad being dead and my not noticing that he wasn't around. Or I have the nightmare about forgetting to feed my horse and then finding him dead from starvation in his stall. Or sometimes I have the one about wolves chasing me across the frozen tundra or the one about crawling into a tunnel and not being able to get out. I am so tired every day from not sleeping, and I keep getting sick.

Today, April 1st

Dad died. He was forty-one. I am seventeen.

July

All day I ride except when I teach a few lessons. Yesterday Counselor actually ran away with me when I was training him for trail riding out on the Mountain Road. He is a racehorse who is just off the track—beautiful! He is a tall, lean thoroughbred whose chestnut coat absolutely glistens in the sunlight. I just gave him his head, and he ran and ran until I knew I had absolutely no say in when he stopped. Eventually, he slowed down to a canter, then a trot, and finally walked. It was great! I felt better than I have in months. I could gallop forever.

Healing

Summer is over, and I am getting my old self back. The drinking has stopped, and I am having a great time with Steve. The other Steve had to go back to Connecticut to get ready to go back to college. Any time I start feeling down, I just close my eyes and think about the best ride of my life. Then I make the ride even better by imagining all the details.

My horse's canter becomes smoother, and he glides over the fences, barely touching the ground in between. I hear the wind rushing past my ears and feel the breeze on my skin. In the distance, I see the next fence, gallop toward it, and relax as my horse soars into the air with his ears pricked forward and every muscle taut. My body and my mind are one with the horse. This is a horse that I have known only in my imagination. He is perfect in every way, integrating the best of each of my favorite horses. Sometimes I go deep into the details of the horse, the way his chestnut coat glistens in the sunlight, how soft he is when I brush my hand over his withers; I feel him nuzzling my neck after we finish our ride and hear him nickering softly. When I open my eyes after a few minutes of thinking all of these thoughts, I always feel better.

Now I have to figure out what to do about the nightmares so I can start getting a full night's sleep. I am going to need plenty of energy because college starts in just a few weeks. I know I made the right choice in going near home. Then I can come home on weekends and help Mom by taking her shopping and doing the other things she needs to take care of. Plus, Steve is in school near my college so we can keep dating, too. By the way, Doug keeps trying to get me to go out with him again, but I am not interested.

Dream Intervention

I think I am figuring out how to stop the nightmares. I started thinking that when I was dreaming, and feeling like I was watching myself in my dream, I could actually step into my dream and manipulate it to my advantage. Rather than succumbing to the fear and disruption of a nightmare, I could take control and change what was occurring into something positive. Recently, I have been experimenting with this concept and am discovering that it is working very well. I expect that I can perfect these techniques over time.

Several nights ago, the wolf dream intruded upon my sleep. Typically, I have found myself pursued over miles of frozen tundra with no assistance in sight. I am always just ahead of the wolves; they are close enough for me to smell their canine earthiness, hear their yelps, and see the saliva drooling from their mouths as they anticipate the taste of their kill. Ahead in the distance I can see a small cabin with a thin trail of smoke coming from its chimney. If I can reach the cabin, I will be able to escape the wolves' jaws. The snow begins and swirls around me, impairing my ability to see either the wolves or the cabin. Continuing to run as fast as I can, through some miracle I find the cabin within my reach. I race to the door, knowing the wolves are just behind me. Plunging toward the door latch, I find it locked. I wake up, drenched in sweat, terrified to sleep again, knowing that the wolves will return.

A few nights later, when the wolf dream came, I stepped into my dream. Instead of running from the wolves I let myself drop back to run with them trusting that, while they were frantic for food, they were not looking at me as a meal but rather as a guide to their food.

As I fell into stride with them, I felt the power of their presence and absorbed their strength. As we raced together, I felt the support of the pack and knew that the wolves could assist me in many ways in my life. The wolves and I moved forward, confident that the cabin would appear as the snow began to swirl around us. Indeed, the cabin lay just ahead. We approached the door with confidence, knowing that inside we would find all that we were looking for. I grasped the latch and found it locked, just as I realized that the lead wolf held a key for me in his jaws. I opened my palm, letting him drop the key into it, and felt him lick the skin of each of my fingers, communicating his love for me. Turning to unlock the door, I found that the key worked perfectly and that the door swung open bathing us all in the warm golden light of the fire. Someone was waiting for me there, but I could not quite make out who it was. I invited the wolves inside to share the meal that awaited them in a large silver feeding bowl. Leaving my lupine friends to their feast, I moved across the room toward the fire and my awaiting host. There, in a rawhide chair by the stone hearth, sat my father—strong, healthy, and looking very content. He welcomed me into an embrace and then sat me down on the soft hearthside rug next to his chair. It was then that I realized that we were in our Sebago cottage and that the chair that he sat in was the same worn leather one that still sits next to our fireplace. The hearth was the same, and the granite chimney held the huge V-shaped hearthstone that marks its center. I drifted along in my dream, feeling comforted and empowered. When I awoke, all of my emotions were positive and I felt very, very good throughout.

The next night, I took myself into the wolf dream, and repeated the previous night's sequence.

All went smoothly and I felt no fear. While I sat with my father by the hearth, the wolves approached us silently and with no malice. Each of the five held a gilt-wrapped gift in his jaw. As the first dropped his gift into my palm, it unwrapped to reveal the gift of perpetual contact with my father through my dreams. The second wolf gave me inner peace and the aware-ness that my father was happy and in a good place. The next wolf came forward bestowing a gift that would lift the remainder of any depression from my spirit, while the fourth gave me the knowledge that if I nurtured my body and engaged deeply with the world and all of its creatures, I would be rewarded with continued good health. And then the fifth wolf stepped forward with his gilt-shrouded gift. As its wrapping fell away, I saw the final treasure. It was the confidence to trust in myself and in the future and to know that, whatever lay ahead, I would find a way to approach it from a positive perspective.

As you can see, I did survive, long into adulthood, and faced challenges that took me deeper into the realm of the natural world and its creatures through athletic endeavors and other experiences. Normal work and family responsibilities and not-so-normal medical episodes presented themselves in the same way that they do for most people. Vigorous outdoor activities, quieter pursuits, and deep engagement in volunteer activities took me through the difficult times and helped me form a way to make the transformational power of our parks, preserves, and the natural world last a lifetime.

Perhaps you would like to reflect now on some of your own childhood experiences and how they contributed to the person you are today. Is there any aspect of what you find there that you would like to feel better about in some way through a visualization that incorporates the world and her creatures?

The healing came for me through a complete immersion in nature that so deeply saturated every fiber of my being that I was able to move through the challenging times more easily. Those were the days before I had regular access to protected green space or even knew that it existed. Instead, the essential wildness of parts of southern Maine drew me in to soothe my body and my mind. Thanks to local land protection efforts and the state-wide efforts of Maine Coast Heritage Trust, The Nature Conservancy, and others, southern Maine continues to hold pockets of conserved lands within its urban environment. Similar efforts exist in every state in our nation where local land trust efforts and community protection of special places ensure that we are able to find the green retreats that we need. On a grander scale are our federal lands— our national forests, national seashores, national monuments, national parks, and Bureau of Land Management lands. All of these areas, as well as the green environment within and around our homes, offer opportunities to soak up images of the world and her creatures. The sights, sounds, smells, and other sensory experiences of these places create a memory bank of material for visualizations that will help us out whenever we need a boost. And, they give us so many chances to reach outside ourselves to have positive impact, even when our own lives feel disrupted.

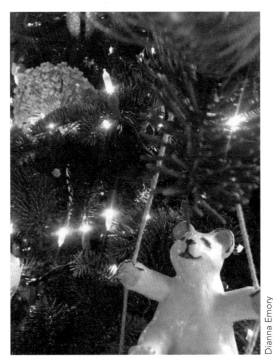

Celebrating another Christmas.

COMMON RECURRING THEMES:
STRESS AND SLEEP DIFFICULTIES

"Over every mountain there is a path,
although it may not be seen from the valley." Theodore Roethke

Relieving Stress

"I am freaking out," says Donna. "I have two kids, my husband has lost his job, I make minimum wage bagging groceries, and now I have breast cancer. I have been trying to finish college by going to night school, and now I can't even count on being able to do that. I am exhausted, I can't even get out the door to get some fresh air, I don't know how to relax, and I know it is going to get worse."

"With a broken hip, at my age I know it is going to take a long time to recover. I have been so addicted to my walks and skis. Sometimes I still do some running. I just don't feel right without it. What am I going to do? And, what about all of the other things I have to worry about?" Sam speaks from his hospital bed, looking toward an uncertain future.

Shariff looks at me frankly, takes a deep breath and lets go. "I feel so guilty about this, but if my stepdaughter moves back in with us, our whole life is going to change. We can't refuse her. She is family, and she is trying to put her life back together. But, I just don't see how we can cope. Privacy in our new little house is going to be non-existent. It is built for two old people. She blasts music constantly and eats everything in sight. I can't deal with this."

"My job is to make my boss and the company look good, but I don't believe in what they are doing. I am caught because I cannot afford to resign. I have to find a way to work this through and deal with all of the stress it is causing me. Can you please help me figure out how to do that? My life and every daylight hour are sucked up by this job," pleads Fred.

Edna is in tears. "Mom is in Oklahoma, and we live in Maine. She is exhibiting signs of Alzheimer's, and I need to help her make some changes. But, my own life feels so overwhelming right now between kids, and work, and trying out a new relationship. How can I cope with all of this as I move my mother east? I need to find a healthy way to get through each day because I am running myself into the ground. I know I am eating all of the wrong things, and I get no exercise. I do not have time to get out of the house except to work."

Why wouldn't you feel stressed? You are moving through a challenging period, you are dealing with a medical situation, someone you love is in crisis, or some other event is feeling overwhelming. Stress is a part of all of our lives, at least from time to time. Sometimes it comes from positive events—marriage, retirement, pregnancy, and outstanding personal achievements all rate high on stress scales. Hans Seyle, an early pioneer of stress research, labeled this kind of stress "eustress." More often, however, we connect stress with the distress of pressure and trauma. When we are faced with a medical or other crisis, as might be expected, our stress index skyrockets. For "senior citizens" over the age of fifty, Stanford University neuroendocrinologist Robert Sapolsky stated, "We now know that aging is about a body that doesn't deal well with stress anymore."[1]

Stress has been defined as a physiological reaction to one's mental activities that causes an internal and external reaction. Among other things, this reaction can lead to a pounding heart, tense muscles, trembling, sweating, nausea, and shortness of breath. Psychological implications include confusion, a shortened attention span, depression, and anxiety. At a critical level, this can result in dysfunction and debilitation, as well as an increase in susceptibility to illness, hormonal imbalance, and suppression of the immune system.

Sheldon Cohen, Ph.D., author of the *Perceived Stress Scale (PSS)*[2], offers a way for you to investigate your own level of stress with this classic stress assessment instrument. Cohen states, "The questions in the PSS ask about your feelings and thoughts during the last month. In each case, you will be asked to indicate how often you felt or thought a certain way. Although some of the questions are similar, there are differences between them, and you should try to treat each one as a separate question. The best approach is to answer fairly quickly. That is, don't try to count up the number of times you felt a particular way; rather indicate the alternative that seems like a reasonable estimate.

The scores on the PSS do not reflect any particular diagnosis or course of treatment. They are meant as a tool to help assess your level of stress. If you have any further concerns about your current well being, please contact your health care provider."

Perceived Stress Scale[2]

For each question, choose from the following alternatives:

0-never 1-almost never 2-sometimes 3-fairly often 4-very often

_____1. In the last month, how often have you been upset because of something that happened unexpectedly?

_____2. In the last month, how often have you felt that you were unable to control the important things in your life?

_____3. In the last month, how often have you felt nervous and stressed?

_____4. In the last month, how often have you felt confident about your ability to handle your personal problems?

_____5. In the last month, how often have you felt that things were going your way?

_____6. In the last month, how often have you found that you could not cope with all the things that you had to do?

_____7. In the last month, how often have you been able to control irritations in your life?

_____8. In the last month, how often have you felt that you were on top of things?

_____9. In the last month, how often have you been angered because of things that happened that were outside of your control?

_____10. In the last month, how often have you felt difficulties were piling up so high that you could not overcome them?

To determine your PSS score, follow these directions:
First, reverse your scores for questions 4, 5, 6, 7, and 8. On these four questions, change the scores like this: 0=4, 1=3, 2=2, 3=1, 4=0
Now add up your scores for each item to get a total.
My total score is _____.

Scores ranging from 0-13 would be considered low stress.
Scores ranging from 14-26 would be considered moderate stress.
Scores ranging from 27-40 would be considered high stress.

There are many things you can do to lower your stress level, even when you are dealing with critical illness or overwhelming life circumstances. Each of these is discussed in greater detail in other portions of this book. When used in concert, they produce a powerful and effective approach to stress management.

Evaluate your eating habits, increasing your consumption of vegetables and fruits and cutting back on meats and fats. Take a look at the charts in this book related to foods. Eliminate or cut back dramatically on the consumption of alcohol, caffeine, sugar, salt, and the use of nicotine. All of these substances exacerbate stress reactions.

Release your feelings through a variety of venting techniques. Talk to your friends and family members or a therapist, **write about your feelings** in a journal, and **express yourself creatively**, perhaps through painting, drawing, clay work, gardening, or dance.

Indulge in a pastime that draws out the quiet beauty within you, reminding yourself that life is a journey, not just a destination. **Find**

opportunities for play and laughter. Enjoy your sexuality.

Express thanks for something each day—to God and the universe, to family members, and/or to friends. Regardless of how difficult things are, there is always something for which to be thankful. Expressions of thankfulness can help to put life in perspective and give others good feelings.

Get yourself outdoors into the world that is provided for you. It is a gift that you can give your body and your mind that will pay you back a thousand times over. Enjoy it in every way that you can, both in quiet contemplation and active engagement. Working up to a minimum of 30 minutes of sweat-producing exercise several days per week can do much to release stress-induced tension. Through snow, sleet, rain, hail, or a beautiful day, walk, run, bike, ski, jump rope, or choose another appealing activity that will give you a physical workout.

If you can't get outdoors choose indoor exercise, even something as simple as going up and down stairs or doing laps inside your house. If you are on a machine, try to position it so that you are looking out a window or at an area where you have houseplants. Investigate some of the nature-related videos that can take you into the natural world while you use a treadmill or other machine. **Tailor your activity level to what is going on in your body** and speed up or slow down accordingly. There is some evidence that says that several bursts of activity throughout the day are more productive than one concentrated activity surrounded by inactivity, so consider trying this approach. We just need to keep moving as much as we can in whatever way works for us at a given point in time!

If you are in medical crisis, follow your doctor's orders and listen to your own mind and body. I am reflecting now on a major injury when I planted my leg through a Virgin Gordan cattle guard and fell at a right angle. Told that there was nothing wrong and I should take pain pills, I threw out the pills and, as soon as I could stand it, dragged my leg up the mountains each morning. The afternoons saw me crawling down the beach into the water and trying to swim with one leg, feeling like a complainer because the doctor had said there was nothing wrong with me. The lesson here is don't always believe what the experts say, if your body is telling you something else. An x-ray a month later when we returned home revealed two broken bones and a host of other traumas.

Engage with nature and the world indoors as well. Watch your fish swimming gracefully around their tank. Interact with your family and your friends. Give your plants a warm shower as you examine the details of their beauty. Brush your cat or dog, giving yourself and your pet some of the contact with another living thing that we all crave. Listen to a lecture about a nature-related topic. Do some research about a species you want to know more about. Watch a video that features beautiful scenery and the kind of activities you enjoy. And, of course, **engage in the relaxation techniques** that can transport you through your mind's eye to the natural world that you love.

Incorporate relaxation techniques into your daily routine and experience the sense of cruising in neutral. Choose from or use a combination of: progressive body relaxation, visualization, self-hypnosis, yoga, meditation, or relaxation recordings. Give yourself the gift of 20-30 minutes each day in a deeply relaxed state, offering your body and your mind an opportunity to restore themselves. Regular sessions of these techniques can lower your blood pressure, reduce stress, and help to alleviate pain.

Follow this program for one month, using other suggestions from this book as well, and evaluate how much you have impacted your stress level by using the Perceived Stress Scale again. The chances are good that you will find that you are coping better in even the most difficult of circumstances.

Overcoming Sleep Difficulties

Dark-circled eyes underscoring the validity of his tale, 32-year-old Michael recounts the thirty consecutive nights he has spent lying awake staring at the ceiling. His usual pattern is to fall asleep soundly after going to bed at about 11:00 and then to jolt to full alertness around 2 AM. He focuses on all of the challenges facing him at work and in his personal life and wrestles with each issue. Typically, it is at least two hours before he drifts off to a sound sleep again. At 6 AM, his ringing alarm clock demands that he rise and begin the day.

The last two weeks have been much worse for Michael. He had learned to live with his 2 AM wakefulness, but the shock of losing his job has thrown him into a period of serious insomnia. He has been worrying about keeping up with the demands of work for quite awhile, but he never thought he would be fired. He struggles to get to sleep each night, tossing around until he flits in and out of a fitful sleep. Each time he drifts off, a thought of what job loss might mean startles him to alertness. Everything seems worse during these nighttime hours, and he has a hard time remembering that he has some good, marketable skills. He worries about what changes will need to be made if he can't get another job, about his insurance, and about the pressures on his family. When dawn finally breaks, he struggles out of bed, exhausted, depressed, and ill-equipped to face a day of trying to find work. Michael's responsibilities have not changed. He has financial obligations and a family to care for. His wife has a minimum wage job, and they need his salary to survive. He is angry and overwhelmed at having his life disrupted by this unanticipated job loss and worries constantly about how he is going to manage. Nighttime anxiety and loss of sleep are draining him of the energy he needs to get through each day. In order to cope, he has developed a pattern of napping for two hours in the afternoon before going to his children's evening events.

We talk a bit about any other changes in the way Michael has been operating since his boss let him know that his position was being cut. He reveals that he has started having a few drinks each evening before bed to help him relax and that he has been too tired most mornings to get out for his usual walk.

Most of us have known the frustration of sleep disruption and many of us are familiar with real insomnia. Once a pattern of poor sleep begins to emerge, it is easy to go into a panic about how many hours we are getting, spending part of the "2 AM Terror" time worrying about how to get in enough hours to manage the next day. When we are facing illness or other crises, it is even more critical that we sleep well. Unfortunately, we are also more inclined to wake and worry. It can be quite a vicious circle. This is what is happening for Michael, in addition to his concerns about his job loss.

How can we help Michael and ourselves to manage this very important issue? First, let's look at what Michael can do, or what we could do in a similar situation, to immediately improve the chances of getting a good night's sleep. Creating a comforting environment that is well-ventilated, dark, and designated for sleep is an important start. Earplugs and white noise from a fan can help to block out distracting sounds.

We know that alcohol precipitates sleep disruption, often giving the consumer a false sense of falling into restful sleep, only to wake a few hours later unable to relax. The healthiest thing we can do is to throw out the window the idea that alcohol in any way positively impacts sleep patterns, getting rid of it during periods of stress or insomnia. The initial sedation that alcohol offers promises sleep disruption later on. Despite the fact that a fine glass of wine or a good rum punch may be a treat, alcohol is really not a great buddy. If you want a drink, have one occasionally, realizing that you may pay for it at 2 or 3 AM.

In Michael's case, he immediately began to cut back on the alcohol, limiting himself to a drink two nights a week. He was not a smoker and was not inclined to eat sweets. Caffeine, however, was a substance he used throughout the day. In order to reduce anxiety and minimize sleep disruption, Michael gradually cut his coffee intake to two 8-ounce cups prior to noon. He was given this information obtained from the Center for Science in the Public Interest:

Substance	Caffeine Content
Black Coffee (12 oz.)	260 mg.
Black Tea (8 oz.)	30-80 mg.
Soda (12 oz.)	30-70 mg.
Dark Chocolate (1.45 oz.)	20 mg.

(Recommended Maximum Daily Allowance for Healthy Adults is 400 mg. of caffeine.)

If you are having trouble sleeping, take a look at caffeine and sugar consumption as sleep-disrupters. Consider limiting or eliminating them. Any caffeine consumption should be minimal and is less disruptive to sleep if it ceases by noon. Desserts and treats consumed at lunch are much less likely to impact sleep than those at dinner. Nicotine is recognized as a sleep-disrupter as well, giving us one more reason not to use it. Also, avoid loading up on a huge meal in the evening. Eat well and in reasonable quantity, making sound nutritional choices that will help to strengthen your body so that it is better prepared to cope with stressors.

Many of the foods that help to induce sleep are right out of our green environment: leafy green vegetables, bananas, pineapples, tofu, roasted soybean foods, beans, asparagus, lentils, and avocados. The post-turkey dinner discussion of the sleep benefits of tryptophan, an amino acid that produces niacin and creates serotonin, is a conversation in which most of us have participated. To encourage relaxation, sleep, and mood stability, boost serotonin production by consuming pumpkin seeds, nuts, tofu, cheese, roasted soybean foods, or turkey. Thiamin (Vitamin B1), which is found in sunflower seeds, salmon, and trout, also helps improve your sleep. Beans, lentils, spinach, avocado, and asparagus contain folate (Vitamin B9), which gives you daytime energy and nighttime sleep.

Exercise is important for releasing tension and increasing fitness. It also can dramatically impact the quality of our sleep. Maintaining a regular exercise pattern is particularly helpful while aging and during stressful periods, even if it means adapting our routine to the demands of illness. Without pushing yourself to exhaustion, give your body a gift of exercise even when it is not at its healthiest. Exercise outdoors, in the green environment, is well-documented as being much more beneficial than indoor exercise[100, 101, 102, 103, 104, 105]. In this era, physicians affiliated with the Green Scripts phenomena, like my friend Dr. Perry Robinson, are writing prescriptions for outdoor exercise as a part of patient treatment plans. This approach has its roots in the 1920s when outdoor enthusiasts including Columbia University's Dr. George Meylan, a physician and president of the American Physical Education Association, purported that outdoor engagement amplified the effects of exercise. Research in Japan's World Heritage Site, Yakushima, and other Japanese forests compared forest walking to treadmill use and urban walking, confirming the increased value of outdoor exercise, as have numerous other studies. As a trail runner, my mind drifts away as I trot along wooded paths that stretch to open vistas of lakes, mountains, and the sea. The scent of evergreens and seaweeds mixes with the feeling of pine needles beneath my feet, the views, and the endorphin-inspired high that fills me with satisfaction. Some of this can come from runs on city streets or on a machine—the endorphin-release, at least—but whenever available, the most natural space around is the one I choose.

The return for an investment in any exercise—even the treadmill or the sidewalk—is more energy, less tension, more restful sleep, and a body better-equipped to deal with whatever it faces. Grab what you can when you can. Do whatever feels appropriate at a particular point in time. For Michael, that meant getting out for his daily walk. Bear in mind, if you are into aerobic activities, that doing them right before bedtime can push one into alertness and disrupt sleep. Save the aerobic exercise for other hours and instead take a warm bath, which can improve both sleep quality and quantity, just before going to bed. I nearly forgot to mention that Michael also added the exercise-incentive of a new rescue dog that needed to go outside each morning and evening. Those pets have many purposes. Do you need one?

The temptation to begin taking naps to make up for poor sleep is hard to resist. A relaxing break in the day can be very important. But, rather than give in to naps on their own, we can gain more benefit through learning relaxation techniques that will help to boost our energy during the day and relax us enough to get to sleep at night. We address how to do this in this book. Of course, if we are ill or recovering from surgery, our bodies may need extra sleep whenever it occurs in order to help us rebuild. In the typical course of life, however, naps in the late afternoon or evening can push us into disrupted nighttime sleep. Rather than succumbing to naps that can alter our sleep patterns, it can be effective to begin using a 20-30 minute relaxation technique or a recorded tape for a boost. You will find a download of a relaxation exercise on my website and scripts in this book.

Wakefulness and sleep disruption can sometimes be eliminated if we settle down for sleep a little later than usual. Engaging in an evening activity that keeps us alert, going to bed an hour later than normal, and setting the alarm for our usual waking time for a few days in a row often helps to compress sleep time and reduce sleep disruption.

If worries are a part of what is making it hard to have a restful night's sleep, it is important to vent these problems during the day. Talking to friends, family, or a therapist can offer successful venting. Writing about the issues and how we plan to deal with each of them can also be very effective. When we are ill, gaining a sense of control through becoming an active part of our treatment team can also go a long way toward helping us to relax. Repetitive worrying while trying desperately to sleep is non-productive. It can be very helpful to get up, write down the worries to attend to the next day, engage in a quiet activity for a half hour or so, and then go back to bed. A preventive approach is to set aside 15 minutes each day to expel worries. Write down your worries and some ways you can impact them. Then, if you wake up and worry, tell yourself that you are already working on the problems.

Sometimes our worries can be so significant that they manifest themselves as nightmares. One of the most effective ways of reducing or eliminating nightmares is through the use of systematic desensitization. Begin by writing down the nightmare in as much detail as you can recall. Do this while you are in a relaxed setting and condition. Then re-write the nightmare, transforming the details to make them friendly and non-threatening. Practice visualizing the new script while you are in a relaxed state. If the nightmare recurs, try stepping outside it, altering it to the new script and relaxing confidently. Without realizing that I was engaging in dream manipulation and lucid dreaming, as a child I transformed my recurrent nightmares into positive experiences. The vicious and hungry wolves that had terrified me for years became my guides as I became their caregiver. Eventually, they led me to a visit with my deceased father and to a much more peaceful life space. Sounds weird? Well, it worked.

The first thing to do if you have trouble getting to sleep is to not try to force it. Instead, do something relaxing like reading a really boring book until you feel tired. For me, that would be something like *121*

Reasons to Re-Learn Calculus. Sleep onset difficulties, as well as sleep maintenance problems, can also be lessened or eliminated through the use of deliberate focusing and progressive relaxation techniques. Our grandmothers' suggestion that we try counting sheep is not silly at all. Focusing on anything other than the problem at hand can help us to be more relaxed. Counting sheep, counting backwards from 1,000, or counting horses jumping over fences, the way I did as a child, can all result in drifting off to sleep.

Progressively relaxing parts of our body is also very effective. Use the download on my website or the script for progressive relaxation from this book, create your own visualization and go deep into its details, or simply focus on telling each part of your body to relax. Begin with the top of your scalp; move over your face, sides and back of your head, and the cords of your neck; go down through your chest, abdomen, and pelvis; down again through your shoulders, upper back, lower back, and buttocks; down each arm all the way to the ends of your fingers; and down each leg to the ends of your toes. The chances are good that this exercise alone will help you to fall asleep. More specific instruction is included in this book's chapter on visualization.

It is important to note that many of us will at some point be offered medication to assist us with sleep disorders. The media bombards us with this "easy" solution and too many physicians offer prescriptions before considering non-drug alternatives. This is not to say that a sedative following surgery is inappropriate or that in extreme cases medication should not be considered. All sedatives, however, are habit-forming over time and complicate any attempt to pursue holistic approaches. Melatonin, a hormone secreted by the pineal gland that activates the physiological processes that promote sleep, has been shown to be helpful in dealing with jet lag and shift workers' sleep problems. Melatonin is sometimes used in the treatment of sleep disorders, but for me, there is insufficient evidence of its effectiveness to recommend it with confidence.

So, have we solved Michael's problems? We certainly haven't found him a new job. It is likely, however, that we have given him some tools that will help him to recover a healthy night's sleep, incorporate these

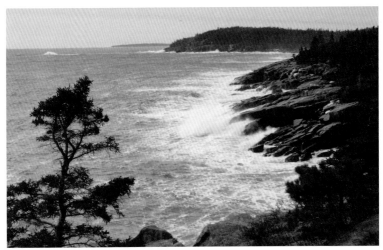

Ben Emory

Lives, like Waves, Have Their Ups and Downs.

approaches into his life plan, and ensure him that, during stressful periods, he knows how to encourage restful sleep. Beginning by helping Michael to get some sleep is a start. Now, we need to help boost his confidence in himself, put depression behind him, and get on with life. That is another story.

CASE STUDIES

"Just living is not enough…one must have sunshine,
freedom, and a little flower."
Hans Christian Anderson

An amputee runs a marathon. A blind woman walks two miles with her dog to her volunteer job teaching calculus to students, and reads their texts in Braille. A physician leaves her country, comes to the United States, and goes to medical school all over again before performing life-saving surgeries. How many times have you looked at someone else's life experience and thought, "If he or she did that, I can get through my challenge!"

A group of case studies of individuals who have faced medical and psychological challenges is presented for your contemplation. All were encouraged to employ cognitive-behavioral approaches to augment their care, including time outdoors interacting with nature; indoor engagement with the natural world; other enrichment opportunities; and adjustments in diet, exercise, and relationship development. Presenting issues include: factors related to aging, the sometimes overwhelming nature of work and responsibilities, stress, cancer, multiple sclerosis, coping with responsibilities related to another's crisis, anxiety, depression, sleep disorders, caffeine toxicity, and other concerns.

Although details have been dramatically altered and names are fictitious, the following case studies are illustrative of some of my professional work. They demonstrate how engagement with the natural world and its creatures can be combined with traditional therapy, visualization, relaxation techniques, appropriate diet, exercise, volunteerism, enrichment activities, and support system development to assist us in coping with life's challenges, as well as in living a healthier life in general. Perhaps you will find these case studies inspirational and helpful as you address your life needs.

Angela

Angela, a slight ten-year-old blonde, was bought to my office by her parents. Angela had been diagnosed with a childhood cancer and was about to undergo chemotherapy. She was experiencing a great deal of trouble getting to sleep each night. In addition, her sleep was frequently disrupted by terrifying nightmares.

A successful student and athlete, Angela was a popular and talented member of her fourth grade class. Her friends and their parents had rallied around her at the time of her diagnosis and offered a strong support system. Thanks to a sensitive teacher, Angela and her classmates were able to openly discuss her situation. At the time that I first saw her, she had missed little school but was unable to participate in the sports that she loved. Her local Y had named her the honorary manager of the swim team and encouraged her to continue to be involved with the team as much as she liked.

Angela's parents were young professionals who were devastated by the illness of their only child. Their first reaction was to immediately relocate to a city near a major cancer research hospital where their daughter could receive cutting-edge treatment. Despite this initial response, they soon realized the importance of maintaining as much consistency as possible in all of their lives. Fortunately, Angela's physicians at her regional hospital and those at the larger oncology research center were willing to structure a treatment program for her that would give her the best of both worlds.

Angela immediately expressed an interest in meeting other children who had been treated for cancer. Television information about camps for children with cancer were her only previous source of knowledge of the illness. We arranged for her to enroll in a children's cancer support group and to meet a young girl who had been successfully treated for her own cancer. This relationship would develop into a lasting friendship. Angela was also interested and excited to learn that I had had my own cancer as a little child and that, regardless, I had gotten to be very old.

We decided to focus on the following issues:

1. elimination of nightmares
2. enhancement of sleep quality

3. instruction in visualization to maintain stomach comfort, provide relief during treatment, and combat cancer.

Angela left my office with my white and fluffy stuffed toy, Beddy Bear, and a small tape player tucked safely inside Beddy's pocket. She would take him to bed with her each night, turn on the tape, and, hopefully, drift off to a sound, undisrupted sleep. If she happened to wake during the night with a nightmare, she could use the tape again. Beddy's tape was one where I had included imagery to dispel nightmares and enhance sleep quality. The approach was based on the one I had used as a child to relieve my own nightmares. I recorded a second tape for Angela to address chemotherapy-related issues. She could take Beddy Bear and this tape to her chemo appointments and also use the approach between sessions.

Because of Angela's keen interest in swimming, we would also incorporate swimming-related imagery into her program to assist her in focusing her thoughts elsewhere during difficult periods—whether at night or in connection with chemotherapy. Angela's parents would be an active part of her treatment and would learn to use relaxation approaches with her. They would also elect to use the techniques to manage their own anxiety and fatigue.

A lover of animals, Angela's counseling was further enhanced through interaction with Chiclet, one of my most trusted horses. While brushing and working with Chiclet, Angela spoke to him of her many worries about her illness. Through me, Chiclet spoke back to her in a reassuring manner. Climbing into the saddle and learning to ride was an empowering experience for her and helped her to feel confident that, if she could master this new skill, she could also be a very strong part of her treatment team.

To keep the animals, swimming, and the nature that she loved in her life—even during difficult periods that could lie ahead—Angela's father filmed and created a video library of her activities. Her mother began to collect little porcelain animals for her, and she and her mother carefully planted a large terrarium where the animals could play.

Throughout her treatment, the many sessions I had with Angela and her parents saw her moving relatively smoothly through the process. Her nightmares and sleep disorder were eliminated. Chemotherapy provided its ups and downs, but it did not produce severe distress. When I last saw her, she went off with Beddy Bear happily in tow. My understanding is that she has done well over the years.

Roberta

Reviewing Roberta's file, I read with a sinking feeling that her primary site breast cancer had spread. At age 47, she was about to begin another chemotherapy round, this time with a stronger drug than the last. Roberta had been referred to me by her oncologist, who knew of my success in working with aversive anticipatory reactions to chemotherapy.

Roberta's therapeutic focus would be on eliminating the nausea and vomiting she experienced when reminded in any way of chemotherapy. Her past reaction was not only to the chemical that had entered her body, but also to specific environmental stimuli. The latest attack had occurred upon seeing her infusion nurse in the local grocery store. Despite the fact that she had not recently had chemotherapy, Roberta was overcome by severe nausea and exited the store just in time to relieve herself in the parking lot. As this round of chemo drew closer, she found herself unable to drive past the hospital where the therapy was administered without being sick. She was already convinced that, when her chemo began, she would be violently ill throughout the treatment period, in addition to continuing with the very unpleasant anticipatory reaction.

Roberta's fear of and reaction to the thought of another round of chemotherapy was mentally and physically debilitating. She was terrified at the thought of spending the next several weeks vomiting in response to the chemo, in addition to being humiliated by her anticipatory reaction. Each night her sleep was disrupted by nightmares about chemotherapy and cancer. She awoke in a high state of anxiety, heart pounding and feeling ill. Her days were spent in a state of exhaustion. She was unable to go to work or to continue with her normal family responsibilities. Fearing anticipatory attacks of nausea, she was reluctant to go outside her house where she might encounter something that would remind her of chemotherapy and trigger an attack. Her only joy was in planning for her spring garden. For Roberta, her treatment felt nearly as bad as the illness.

Roberta entered my office with some apparent trepidation. Her resigned and worn expression was reinforced by the dark circles under her sleepless eyes. As we greeted one another and she sank into the sofa, she dissolved into sobs. We talked about her cancer history, her treatment, and the debilitating nature of her worries. Together, we developed a treatment plan to help her through her chemotherapy and illness. Her role in the treatment team was emphasized, despite the fact that she stated that there was nothing she could do. Roberta identified her primary concerns as:

1. fear of chemotherapy and the related problems with fatigue, nausea, and vomiting
2. fear of anticipatory nausea and vomiting
3. anxiety
4. insomnia
5. depression.

She listened with interest as I described some of the things we could do immediately to impact the way she was feeling. Underlying the plan was the need to empower Roberta and help her realize that she could play an important role in her own treatment. Currently, she felt out of control, swept along in a tide of doctors, symptoms, treatments, and cancer.

As an immediate intervention, I did a relaxation training session with Roberta, incorporating instruction in deepening techniques. Into the session, I built imagery related to the gardens and flowers that she loved. This session resulted in Roberta's feeling more relaxed and in control and left her with an understanding of how to bring on the relaxation response. She also understood that she could use progressive body relaxation and visualization at any time to lower her anxiety level, relieve fatigue, or to relax into sleep during periods of insomnia.

Roberta reported on her intake of caffeine, alcohol, and sugar; described her exercise patterns; and acquainted me with her health history. Although much of this information was available through her physician's file, it was important for Roberta to directly convey her perspective.

Roberta acknowledged that she drank four cups of coffee each morning to get going. She did not drink alcohol. Her primary sugar intake was a few rich chocolates with an espresso each night. We discussed the implications of this level of caffeine ingestion. Roberta was surprised to learn that caffeine could stay in her system for many hours after she went to bed and that the chocolate was giving her an additional caffeine jolt. The connection between caffeine and her anxiety was also illustrated. Although coping with cancer was an obvious source of anxiety, Roberta understood that her caffeine intake was exacerbating her symptoms and increasing her level of anxiety. Together we constructed a chart that would help her to gradually cut back on caffeine and minimize withdrawal symptoms. She thought that she would look forward to a reward when she reached her goal and made plans to buy an especially lovely peony for her garden.

Because Roberta had essentially given up all exercise, she was encouraged to get back out into the garden and to take a daily walk, first on her own expansive property and later on a portion of one of Acadia National Park's easier carriage roads. Roberta said that she was going to immediately get herself outdoors on days when she felt well and return to her walks in the Park. She chose to alternate between the Eagle Lake carriage road and the Witch Hole Pond/Paradise Hill carriage road, starting with half hour walks, with the hope of building up to regularly walk the entirety of one or the other of those 6.5 mile loops. She agreed to do this as a way to spend some time with her friend, who was already on a weight-loss walking program. We also agreed to hold some of our therapy sessions within Acadia National Park, either walking or finding a comfortable place to relax and engage in some visualization experiences.

In the event that circumstances interfered with her walks, we developed a plan for enrichment activities that would maintain Roberta's contact with the natural world that included enhancing her indoor green space and researching plants and landscaping plans.

During a visualization session that included imagery related to systematic desensitization, we focused on reducing or eliminating Roberta's conditioned response to reminders of chemotherapy. We also worked on alleviating the nausea and vomiting associated with infusions. To help Roberta change her image of chemotherapy as an enemy, imagery related to her gardens and her walks in Acadia National Park, with details of the plants she encountered, was incorporated. This would help her view the chemo as a positive part of her treatment team. Healing imagery was also included. Instruction in self-hypnosis was reinforced in the session. Upon waking each day, Roberta agreed to listen to a 35-minute relaxation therapy tape targeting positive feelings, good health, and increased energy.

Roberta left the session feeling more in control of her life and with some new skills that could help her alleviate some of her discomfort. We worked together for three more sessions and one at her home just prior to her first infusion. Roberta's anticipatory response to chemo was extinguished. She experienced some mild nausea on the day following two of her infusions and one episode of vomiting, a considerable change from her last round of chemo when she experienced severe nausea with vomiting after each session. Roberta gradually replaced her coffee with decaf or tea over a two-week period. She began having her chocolate snack after lunch rather than dinner. She used progressive body relaxation and self-hypnosis once a day for twenty minutes; listened to her relaxation tape each afternoon during her low energy period; began taking a daily 45-minute walk with her friend; and succeeded in eventually easily walking a 6.5 mile loop. Roberta was one of the most compliant patients with whom I have ever worked. The impact of her strong role in the treatment process brought good results. She found that her periods of anxiety decreased significantly and that, when she did experience anxiety, she was able to lower it through using visualization techniques.

Although Roberta's cancer was not cured, she experienced much less discomfort during her treatments and returned to a normal life where she was working and fully engaged with family and friends. Future rounds of chemotherapy were not a problem for her.

Hugh

Hugh arrived in my office in a high state of anxiety. Recently released from inpatient treatment for Generalized Anxiety Disorder because his insurance ran out, Hugh was in a highly agitated state. Wringing his hands, pacing around the room, and frequently twitching, he reported that he could not control his panic and irritability, that he kept thinking that he was going to die from a heart attack, and that he had lost his job because he could not concentrate or complete assigned tasks. Our intake interview revealed that Hugh had not eaten since the night before and had consumed six cups of coffee before his appointment. His last intake of beverage or food had been coffee and cake at 11 PM. Further inquiry revealed that Hugh typically had twelve to fourteen cups of coffee each day, often accompanied by sweets. He ate hotdogs with cola for lunch and takeout food for dinner in the late afternoon, followed by cola, sweets, and then his pre-bedtime snack of more coffee and sweets. Hugh was approximately 150 pounds overweight. He got no exercise, used no relaxation approaches, was single with no friends and no pets, and said he had little interest in anything other than the technical aspects of computers and watching TV shows. Hugh stated his primary concerns as:

1. an inability to control shaking and twitching
2. loss of his job
3. an inability to concentrate or complete jobs
4. fear of dying from a heart attack
5. lack of friends because of his irritable and explosive temperament.

It wasn't easy to convince him, but Hugh was eventually able to see the parallels between some of his problems, his sugar consumption, and caffeine toxicity. Because he had undergone a complete physical evaluation before our meeting, his symptoms had been attributed to mental health issues, and he had been declared physically healthy, aside from his obesity. Hugh agreed to begin gradually cutting back on his caffeine and sugar intake. He agreed to begin attending Overeaters Anonymous to help him to develop a healthier diet and a support system. He met with me once a week in an outdoor setting to have a therapy walk and once a week in the office to work on relaxation techniques. After four weeks, he reported forming friendships within his OA group as well as a significant reduction in his anxiety level.

At six weeks, one of his new friends accompanied him to the local animal shelter to pick out a dog. Hugh then began taking daily walks with his dog and began helping out at the shelter, where he was given the volunteer job of dog walking, which he loved. We talked about how caring for a dog could help him to learn to take better care of himself and to transfer the positive way he related to animals to similar interactions with people.

At eight weeks he was down to two cups of coffee a day and one dessert a day. He used a relaxation tape upon waking and in the late afternoon. All symptoms of an anxiety disorder had vanished: no twitching, no shaking, no heart pounding, less irritation with others, fewer worries about dying of a heart attack, and increased ability to concentrate and complete tasks. Although he was still unemployed, he looked forward to summer when more positions would be available in his community. By mid-summer he had established an active private computer repair business and was regularly seeing friends from the animal shelter and his OA support group. His dog walks were leading him to all parts of Acadia National Park, and he had lost 50 pounds. He had given up all sweets and caffeine and was having no trouble with anxiety or its symptoms. At last report, Hugh was leading a fulfilling life and functioning well.

Byron

Byron, a burly married man in his mid-fifties, was referred to me by his physician for treatment of depression and assistance with the side effects of prostate surgery. Two years earlier, Byron had undergone successful surgery for early stage prostate cancer. His prognosis for a full recovery was excellent. Although his surgeon felt that there was no medical reason for lingering side effects, Byron continued to experience erectile dysfunction. He described his depression as related primarily to his difficulties in sexual performance and his fear of dying before age sixty. He also related that, for much of the time when he was not at work in his job as a secondary school math teacher, he felt exhausted. Consequently, he never engaged in any type of exercise and was reluctant to plan any social engagements.

Byron described his weekends of lying on the sofa, watching television, and slipping in and out of naps. He was also in the habit of drinking ten to fourteen beers over the course of each day. On weekdays, Byron limited himself to two beers before dinner. He drank no other alcohol and stated that he "stuck to beer" because he didn't want to be an alcoholic like his father. Prior to his prostate surgery, Byron's weekend drinking habits had been consistent with the weekday self-imposed limit. When asked where he felt joy in his life, Byron responded, "when thinking about how I used to go fishing." His reply to an inquiry about his purpose in life was "just staying alive" and "thinking of the way things used to be."

Sondra, Byron's wife of twenty-eight years, accompanied him to our sessions. Sondra immediately stated that she was very upset with Byron for wasting his life and not putting his illness behind him. She said she loved him very much and wanted him to start enjoying life again. She described her frustrations with their situation as related primarily to Byron's lack of interest in "doing anything fun." While she missed their formerly satisfying sexual relationship, she was more concerned that Byron had given up all of the activities he had previously enjoyed, many of which they had shared as a couple. These activities included his saxophone playing, their evenings attending musical performances, their daily walks in Acadia National Park, fishing expeditions, and their times with friends. Byron and Sondra had no children and, of their parents, only Byron's eighty-four-year-old mother was still living. Byron's three younger siblings all lived in other parts of the country and were only in sporadic contact. His mother, however, lived in her own home in their community and was a regular visitor to their home. She routinely moved to Byron and Sondra's house on Friday evenings where she could "help to take care of Byron" until he returned to work on Monday morning. Then, back she would go to her own active life. She and Sondra appeared to work together to provide for all of Byron's needs, despite the fact that she also wanted him to put his illness behind him and "get on with his life."

Both Sondra and Byron acknowledged that they shared many wonderful and loyal friends who were "waiting for Byron to recover" so that they could all start enjoying shared activities again.

Byron stated his primary concerns as:

1. sexual difficulties
2. worries about dying
3. depression
4. strengthening his relationship with Sondra.

In order to give Byron a sense of his own role in impacting his treatment, we began by reviewing his food and beverage consumption and his exercise routine. He and Sondra agreed to walk together for 45 minutes each morning and to add a second walk in the afternoons on Saturdays and Sundays. While on their Acadia National Park walks, they elected to begin recording the presence of the birds that they loved and also saw at their home feeders. With excitement, they agreed to begin planning a fishing trip. They both acknowledged that they had been consuming far too many prepared foods and decided to work as a couple to plan a weekly menu that would include healthier foods. We addressed food as fuel and how the birds and animals that they loved used exactly this approach to feeding. Byron and Sondra liked the idea of trying this approach to eating. To provide structure, I helped them to develop a chart and reporting system that would assist them in monitoring their progress related to their diet and exercise.

When we discussed his alcohol consumption in greater detail, Byron admitted that he felt out of control of his weekend beer drinking. He expressed surprise that beer could relate to alcoholism and panicked at the thought that he could be following in his father's footsteps. He then went on to say that he actually knew he was doing this and that his father had died at age 58 from a heart attack after a bout with prostate cancer that had been followed by increased drinking. Byron acknowledged that he was convinced that he would soon meet the same fate as his father. After a lengthy discussion of treatment approaches and self-help programs, he expressed interest in joining an Alcoholics Anonymous group as a way of establishing a broader support system and eliminating his beer drinking. He also agreed to a consult with the local outpatient substance abuse treatment center.

To work on his depression, we designed a depression scale for Byron to use on a daily basis to monitor his level of depression during the first month of our weekly appointments. Prior to considering antidepressants, it was important to assess the impact that decreased alcohol consumption, a healthier diet, a regular exercise routine, and therapy could have on his depression.

To address their sexual concerns, Byron and Sondra would meet with me on a weekly basis. Part of his treatment would involve visualization and systematic desensitization to focus on alleviating his erectile dysfunction, which appeared to connect to his fear of having a heart attack and dying. He and Sondra would also work in a structured program to gradually increase their level of intimacy. They would both use creative visualization and charting as a part of this process.

Byron and Sondra also committed to a minimum of one social engagement a week for the first month of treatment, with a goal of reconnecting with their friends.

Byron's fear of dying was rooted in the similarities between his and his father's lives. Regular physical exams did not help to dispel his fears. His mother's role in enabling Byron's slow recovery also paralleled the manner in which she cared for his father during the last few years of his life. Traditional talk therapy was used to address these issues. Byron's mother was brought into some of the sessions.

Cognitive-behavioral techniques, including visualization, charting, and guided imagery, were also employed to help Byron let go of his fear of dying and gain a sense of active participation in where his life was heading. As Byron and Sondra increased their time walking and birding in Acadia National Park, they developed a keen interest in the plants that lived there as well. While challenging one another to recall Latin names of each species, they were inspired to create a wild garden in their own back yard. As winter approached, they delighted in bringing bits of moss, berries, and ferns into their home to build small terrariums. Spring saw a fishing trip to Grand Teton National Park.

Despite two setbacks related to non-compliancy, after eight months in treatment Byron had achieved all of his goals, and he was symptom-free. His depression had abated without the use of anti-depressants. He and Sondra were maintaining a healthy diet, and Byron had ceased his beer drinking. He continued in an AA support group and a counseling program at the hospital outpatient substance abuse program. Byron's erectile problems dissipated over time, with normal functioning returning after eight months. He and Sondra had strengthened their relationship in many ways, were once again enjoying time with their friends, and were spending quality time with his mother that focused on shared interests rather than Byron's illness. Six years later, he had experienced no further problems with cancer. Neither had he exhibited any problems with his heart.

Byron's case is included here to illustrate how cancer can sometimes be a precipitating catalyst for the development of other problems. With appropriate intervention, including engagement with the natural world and its creatures, many difficulties related to mental health concerns can be alleviated.

Susan

Susan was devastated by her breast cancer diagnosis. A 68 year-old single woman with a long history of depression and abuse, she had spent years involved in many different therapies, including a ten-year relationship with an unlicensed "counselor" who seemed to make no progress in assisting her, but had happily collected his fees. Susan had been off and on a number of anti-depressants over the years, but tended to be non-compliant. She was resistant to further medication, saying that it made her feel "weird and more out of control."

After her recent move to our community, I had taken Susan on as a client and had been using cognitive-behavioral strategies to help her gain some control over her situation. She had proved to be very receptive to relaxation therapy and had begun using related audiotapes on a regular basis. She had made adjustments in her diet and exercise patterns and was pleased to be both dropping weight and feeling better. As a part of her treatment, we had examined her interests in search of an activity that would give her an outward focus and help her to feel that she was doing something productive. An animal lover and dog owner, she had begun volunteering at the local animal shelter and was thrilled with her success at finding placements for the needy dogs and cats. Each day she spent two hours walking dogs on the wooded trails near the shelter, studying trees and plants along the way. She reinforced these observations online, learning more about the natural world. Susan's life had taken a positive turn in many ways, and she was feeling very encouraged about the future. Then a routine mammogram turned up a suspicious lump that proved to be malignant.

Susan was shattered by her diagnosis, but anxious to proceed with the recommended lumpectomy and get on with her life. She asked me if I would use clinical hypnosis to assist her in preparing for her surgery. Susan's surgeon was a well-respected physician, who was open to including alternative approaches in her treatment. He had previously welcomed me into the operating room and allowed me to stand next to his patient throughout the surgery. From this vantage point, I could continue the hypnosis throughout the surgery and also keep a reassuring hand on the patient's shoulder or forehead.

Susan's surgery was scheduled for two weeks from the time of our meeting, giving us the opportunity to have three more appointments before her surgery. I would then join her at the hospital, where we would begin a hypnosis session in the pre-operative room. I would continue this session throughout her surgery. After her lumpectomy, we would have at least one follow-up visualization session as a part of her regular meetings with me. Beyond that, we would reinforce some of the preliminary suggestions regarding eradication of any stray cancer cells and returning to optimum health.

Susan responded well to the three pre-surgical sessions. Incorporating her own imagery related to her dog walks and plant observations came easily to her. We worked on preparing her body and mind for a pleasant and successful surgical experience. It was stressed that Susan was an important part of the treatment team. Suggestions were made for the following:

1. general relaxation with a positive, interested, and welcoming attitude toward the surgery

2. reduction of blood flow during the surgery

3. the need for less anesthesia due to a pre-surgical hypnotic state

4. a speedy post-operative recovery with little discomfort.

Susan awoke from her surgery feeling relaxed, positive, and confident of an easy recovery. Her physician reported that all had gone very well, there were clean margins, and he anticipated no complications. Susan would receive follow-up radiation.

In the days following her surgery, Susan gained strength quickly. She turned regularly to humorous animal videos that she said got her laughing so hard that she nearly split her stitches. During her recovery, she was pleased to stamp envelopes for the shelter as a way of helping out. Her own dog entertained her and kept her company as she strengthened. Soon Susan returned with enthusiasm to her volunteer activities. She also embarked on an assertive mission to eradicate any future cancer cells. She incorporated taped relaxation sessions with personalized strengthening and cancer-fighting visualizations into her daily routine. These visualizations were based on her paintings, clay work, and drawings. Susan also maintained a healthy diet, began volunteering at the shelter again, and quickly returned to her normal exercise pattern.

Eight years later, Susan remained cancer-free and reported a "fulfilling and happy life." She said that she had become quite an expert at developing her own visualizations and particularly enjoyed inserting imagery related to playing with dogs in fields. She was still volunteering and feeling very good about her contributions. Susan was also building a portfolio of animal paintings for an exhibit and said that she planned to paint pictures of dogs in fields until she was too old to pick up a paintbrush.

Jenny

Jenny, a 26-year-old artist, was referred to me by her physician after she had inquired about mind-body approaches that could be used to enhance the multiple sclerosis treatment process. An awareness of her family history had led to a diagnosis after fatigue and other issues developed. Because Jenny's father and sister had both been diagnosed with

MS, Jenny was not surprised at her diagnosis.

A slim, dark-haired beauty, Jenny had already met with enormous success in her life. Her paintings were being exhibited nationally, and she was in demand at many major galleries. At 26, she was a successful marathon runner, had excelled in competitive swimming at college, and continued to participate regularly in a wide range of athletic endeavors. Although she was single, she had a steady boyfriend whom she planned to marry when he completed his MBA. Jenny's social network was extensive. She regularly entertained and was engaged in a variety of cultural activities. As a volunteer art therapist ten hours a week in a children's psychiatric hospital, Jenny felt satisfied that she was using her artistic ability in a way that would help others.

Jenny stated that she had "always expected" that she would have to deal with multiple sclerosis at some point in her life. While she was certainly not ecstatic about her diagnosis, she implied that she viewed this part of her life as something that she could work with, although she acknowledged the uncertain course of the illness.

During our initial session, Jenny identified several areas where she would like my assistance:

1. focus on maintaining her body's fitness level through a review of her diet and exercise regimen
2. instruction in relaxation techniques for use on a daily basis to combat fatigue
3. instruction in creative visualization techniques that she could incorporate into her daily routine to help with multiple sclerosis side effects and enhance response to treatment.

A review of Jenny's diet and exercise routine revealed that she was taking very good care of herself. She chose to abandon her one glass of wine a day and her cup and a half of coffee, stating that she no longer wanted to put anything into her body that didn't "have a productive purpose."

As we talked about her support system and opportunities for venting, Jenny chose to immediately join a support group for MS patients. She indicated a desire to "help the group" and enthusiastically embraced the idea of volunteering to do some art-related work with the members.

Because of her excellent visualization skills and her artistic inclinations, we decided that she would use clay and fingerpaints to depict what she viewed as her "war on MS," and that she could assist others in this capacity as well.

Jenny found her first experience with progressive relaxation and visualization intriguing and exciting. She requested two appointments a week for assistance in building these techniques and self-hypnosis into her life.

Within a week, she had begun using her relaxation tape on a daily basis, was practicing self-hypnosis, had eliminated her coffee and wine, and had met with the MS support group. A portfolio of finger paintings depicting her MS war accompanied her. The gray, amorphous blob was clearly being defeated by a bold and strong army of vibrantly colored "body helpers."

For strengthening, Jenny and I designed a tape that incorporated her painting imagery as well as other suggestions. She declared herself as feeling positive—ready to "get on with the rest of life." This life would also include an aggressive daily visualization to combat any future exacerbations. Several more sessions with Jenny saw her continuing in her very assertive and positive approach. Two years later, she had remained on a medical plateau, had not experienced any further debilitating exacerbations, and was working as an art therapist in an oncology setting. This is not a suggstion that visualization cured Jenny's MS, but it might have made things easier.

6

VENTURING FORTH TO ENGAGE DEEPLY WITH THE NATURAL WORLD:
from Your Own Environment to the Larger Community

THE LAND
"Wilderness is not luxury but a necessity of the human spirit."
Edward Abbey

THE SKY
*"For my part, I know nothing with any certainty,
but the sight of the stars makes me dream."*
Vincent Van Gogh

THE WATERS, FRESH AND SALT
*"The sea is everything. It covers seven-tenths of the globe.
Its breath is pure and healthy. It is an immense desert,
where man is never lonely, for he feels life stirring on all sides."*
Jules Verne

Forming a symbiotic relationship with the natural world can begin wherever you find yourself right now. Scan your interior environment and zero in on the first green thing that you see. For me, it is the orchid sitting on my desk. Its blooms are past, but its leaves are fresh and tiny buds promise rebirth. Two roots stick out from the pot, little poking caterpillar nubs searching for something beyond their home, seeming to beckon to me to come closer. Hmm. There seem to be long, white cat hairs on the orchid's leaves, indicating that something went on here between fauna and flora last night.

What particular bit of green life are you seeing inside your home, and what notes can you make about its appearance? Start with what you see directly, observing what detail you can. If you have a magnifying glass or a botanist's loop (available from Bausch and Lomb), take a really close look. Record all that you can see. How are you feeling as you look at your plant? Do you feel a connection to it? (If you do not have a plant somewhere in your house, please invest in one orchid. You can buy them for under $20 at Home Depot, and they will earn their keep for years. These miraculous plants are one of the easiest with which to establish a relationship and are simple to care for. Just ask "Ryan the Orchid Guy" at Ryan@OrchidsMadeEasy.com.)

Are you hearing any sounds of life as you study your plant? Eliminate whatever man-made noise you can and really listen for a few minutes. What natural sounds can you hear, regardless of the human-made ones that may be ever-present? Try zeroing in on them in the same way you did the visual details. The rain is pattering against my windowpanes, offering up sustenance to spring bulbs and perennials, and I can hear a crow calling, despite the fact that traffic sounds are also evident.

Does your nose detect any fragrances? Inhale deeply, close your eyes for a minute, and take a deep sniff. What do your olfactory senses find? The scent of coffee might block out everything else here, but I know that is a gift of the natural world as well.

How about a living creature within your home? If you have a pet, go deep into the details of the creature you see, and touch that animal, too. If you have no pet, look around for some other living creature. I know where a ghost spider is living in my laundry room, as well as a ladybug that I saw on a plant this morning. Either one provides an opportunity for study, but probably does not invite touch. We have this fat white kitty who is now snoring as loudly as the pouring rain and begins to purr loudly as I stroke her silky fur. That would be the same white fur that typically coats every pair of black pants I own. Her details are numerous—soft paws that pat us when it is dinner-time, a pale pink nose, and long-lashed cat eyes that I will remember forever. Is there a way you would like to enrich your interior space through bringing in more plants or animals? One orchid and a couple of fish are a start!

Now choose a favorite window from which you can see something of life outdoors, a place that is ripe for examination and the stimulation of a host of memories. Even if you are looking out at a city street, search for a bit of green or a living thing. As you focus on life outside your window, go deep into the sights, the sounds, and the memories. Then, record where your thoughts have taken you.

In your imagination, how about joining me here in Maine, where the conifers etch their green branches against the sky? From my window, we see three white pines, two spruces, and several small oaks and maples that are beginning to unfurl. The crows are up there in the pines, calling out, probably preparing to check on the status of the phoebes' nests or take more than their share from under the bird feeders around the corner. Their sleek feathers and curious eyes are so familiar, reminding me of a crow from forty years ago who rode daily upon the rump of my daughter's gray pony. Last spring's memorable crow event occurred when they took out apparent anger at a day's lack of seeds. Returning home, we discovered at least twenty tulip heads nipped off cleanly and thrown about. The next morning, we watched the crows confirm their guilt. They were scolded, and we complied with their daily seed allotment. Refocusing on plants, the field below the crows' pines holds patches of trailing arbutus, mayflowers, in full bloom. Although their tiny pink blossoms and leathery leaves await my trip out the door, I can conjure up their fragrance as my fingers type these words, filling my head with more joy than memories of nipped tulips. Can you recall the fragrance of mayflowers or another blossom? Perhaps the thought of lilacs or a sprig of lavender will quickly bring you a memorable scent. Close your eyes, and inhale again.

What is outside your door, and how do you embrace it? Think about that for a minute and make some notes. Rain or shine, we head out the door to delve into the area right around the house. The chickadees' songs call to me, the sweet sound of a thrush beckons, and the drumming of a pileated woodpecker announces his presence. Let's turn back to you. Maybe you would like to go out your door right now to listen carefully for nature's sounds, breathe in her scents, and examine the details of her flora and fauna. Wherever you are, even if it is on a busy city sidewalk, there is likely still a bit of the natural world awaiting your examination. As you take a stroll there, make some more notes of what you find and once again go deep into the detail. Just be careful of where you are going. I did this once, and fell off the steps into the rose bushes.

Near your own home, you are probably familiar with a myriad of community spaces ripe for exploration. If you are not, check out the website for your town or local land trust to find the closest place where you can get away from the din. You might want to go soon to one of those places, walking if possible.

Join me now on a walk to a vernal pool on the edge of a blueberry barren, where I will spend about 15 minutes observing bugs and, hopefully, something else. Up a wooded road we go, into the barrens that stretch as far as we can see. Along the edge, we find the pool and stand silently by, waiting to see what happens. The vegetation is thick and ripe with muck and algae. As a wood frog dives into the pool, we are astounded to see a thin snake moving from the wet leaves down into the depths of the pool. This is a Northern red-bellied snake, one of several local snakes that can survive on land or in water. At the back of this small pool we see a mass of wood frog eggs that can easily be differentiated from salamander eggs. Frogs lay individual clear eggs in masses with the outline of each egg seen within the mass, while salamanders coat their entire egg mass with an additional layer of gel and often attach their egg masses to sticks. Common toads lay their eggs in strings. We do not see toad eggs here, but let's go look them up online later. Did you know that sometimes egg masses can look cloudy due to the genetic makeup of the female, not some ailment? Don't you want to just climb right into that pool with all of these creatures to see what else we can find?

While I sit here in the mud in the vernal pool for a while longer, you might want to immerse yourself in your own community green space and seek the intricacies of life there. If you are unable to get outside, tap your memory for a time when you did venture into a nearby green space and recall what you found there.

As we take our outdoor retreats to the next level, let's focus on the state park systems across our country. With more than 10,230 of them to choose from, there is probably one near you. We especially enjoyed the Florida Panhandle's St. Joseph Peninsula State Park at Cape San Blas that introduced us to sandy scrub trails, fascinating vegetation, rewarding birding, and miles of pristine beaches. How about choosing a state park destination, and increasing your repertoire of flora and fauna encounters therein? If we struck out in our car today, intent on state park visitations, what an adventure we would have had by the time we found number 10,230.

From the state park system, we move to the 56 million acres that have been preserved across the country, thanks to the land trust movement. The Land Trust Alliance (LTA) strengthens land conservation across America by bringing together more than 1000 member land trusts through training, advocacy work, land protection, and an interest in connecting people to the land. These individual land trusts work with donors of land and conservation easements to protect important areas, many of which provide for public access. It has been my good fortune to serve on the Board and the Council of Maine Coast Heritage Trust and to be married to a former executive director of both MCHT and the Land Trust Alliance. Whenever I need a fact check, my personal expert and conservation mentor, Ben Emory, is across the desk writing his own book, *Sailor for the Wild.*

As you can see, we are building our connection to the natural world, branching out from the interior space of our own home to our back-yard, to community resources, to state parks and other protected areas, and then on to our national parks. As we age, encounter medical issues, or are constrained in other ways, we can reverse this order. Through recalling details of green spaces, remembering our activities there, and learning to draw from our memories and our imaginations to build strong sensory images, we find ourselves able to tap all of what we have experienced—even when limited to our interior space. We follow this route, sometimes shoring ourselves up for the future, while other times taking a deep breath before plowing through a challenge. We are facing life head-on and doing all that we can to maximize our benefits from life's peak experiences in order to weather the valleys in a more comfortable manner.

Now, we are going to try the "Where are you today?" approach again, as it gives another opportunity to sink deeply into the world around you, absorbing it for its current value and restorative potential.

What piece of green environment is within your reach so that you can enjoy it and then easily tap its imagery when you want? How do you want to engage with that place today? For me, signs of spring are around as the days grow longer, robins hop along listening for worms, and the eagles with last year's young fly low across the fields. The narcissi are up one inch, a few patches of snow hang on stubbornly, while the rhododendron branches brought indoors in February are in full bloom. This morning, I choose not to stay on land. Rather, it is the bay that draws me to it on this April day that finally feels like springtime.

From the bay, Acadia's mountains line the horizon presenting tempting thoughts of adventures there after this expedition on the water. Acadia holds a multitude of promises. Out on Frenchman Bay, the guillemots have replaced the longtails. We are missing one loon— gone, we fear, to the eagles. Ben saw a big white-headed adult carrying something black and white across the cove last week. They can pick up a small cat, we witnessed years ago, so they can surely carry one of last year's loon babies. Once an endangered species, the bald eagle has recovered in many places, including on Mount Desert Island and in Acadia National Park.

The sun casts a long sparkling path from the east, and the breeze encourages me to head for Hadley Point and the site of the eagles' nest. Do all three live in that nest? And what happens when this year's young are born? Are the adolescents kicked out to make room for their younger siblings? All of those questions can be answered by a few hits on the keyboard, something I find almost as miraculous as spring's rebirth. I am a product of days when all research took place in library stacks and through interlibrary loan. How far we have come technologically, and what intellectually stimulating opportunities there are for us on-line! For now, we want to be outdoors as much as possible, but that world of technological wonders holds promise for those times when old age or illness shuts our door. Right now, a paddle board on Frenchman Bay waits for me.

With the wind on the nose, the chop across the bay has built, but the resistance of it feels good. My view trains on the eagles' nest and how it rests in the crook of the tallest white pine on the point. Why do I never see the eagles making repairs? I know these nests are built to last a lifetime, but there must be some occasional damage from the howling northwest winds—one more thing to learn about at a later time.

Turning and putting the wind at my back, the panorama of sky and water and evergreen shore reveal how available those things are to most of us, regardless of where we find ourselves, thanks to advocates for conservation. In the city, the joy of a Central Park run, replete with pockets of dog parties, gives a positive start to the day. Olmsted knew what he was doing when he strove to create "pleasure gardens" for escape from city pressures. Later, the community or urban park movement was driven by recreational opportunities, particularly pools, playgrounds, and ball fields close to clusters of housing. Many of the early community parks were let go during the mid-1900s, but have since been resurrected. Interesting data from Resources for the Future[37] states that at last survey, in 2009, 85% of urban park directors surveyed indicated an increase in hiking or walking, 90% of park directors surveyed indicated an increase in popularity of dog parks, and 80% of those surveyed indicated an increase in skate park popularity.

As we move from community parks to look at state parks, according to the National Association of State Park Directors, as of 2014 the United States had 10,234 state park units, with 739 million annual visits. "The big boost to state park systems came with the establishment of the Civilian Conservation Corps in 1933. This work relief program put young men between the ages of 17 and 23 to work planting trees, cutting trails and scenic vistas, and constructing picnic areas, campgrounds, cabins, bathhouses, and other facilities…state parks originally focused on preservation rather than recreation. But, beginning in the 1960s, increased demand for recreation fueled development of state park facilities."[38]

By 2015, there were 25,800 protected areas in the United States covering 499,800 square miles, as well as 787 National Marine Protected areas stretching over an additional 490,893 square miles.

As Theresa Pierno, President and CEO of the National Parks Conservation Association, states, "Today's report shows that our national parks are more popular than ever. From the shores of Acadia to the peaks of Rocky Mountain and hallowed ground at Gettysburg, our national parks are dynamic places that people from around the world visit to have once-in-a-lifetime experiences and, as these numbers show, national parks are becoming even more popular."[39] Regarding our national parks, Secretary of the Interior Ryan Zinke stated that 2016 visitation was up 7.7% over the previous record-breaking 2015 rate. The National Park 2016 centennial year saw nearly 331 million visitors to the system.[40] As of 2016, more than 13 billion visits had been made to our national parks since data collection by the National Park Service began in 1904.[41]

Not everyone can travel to a national park. Most of us, however, can get outside into some green area where we feel that we have contact with the natural world and her creatures. At the very least, we have our memories and the ability to delight our senses through creative visualization. What are some of the most available places for your exploration? The deeper your engagement with those natural places and their creatures, the more memories you will create, the more paths you can travel in your mind's eye, and the more promise you will find in making this connection last a lifetime.

We know well the opportunities that exist to use our bodies to take us to magnificent places where we can experience all that the green outdoors holds. Personal immersion in the protected green spaces of our world is readily available, whether we focus on our own environment or reach beyond it.

Together we will explore the two national parks that I know intimately, expanding our horizons beyond our home environment and our state and community lands and waters to the federal lands of which we are all stakeholders. As models for engagement with the natural world, I have included some detailed information about two of our ocean-connected national parks, Acadia National Park and Virgin Islands National Park. Use what is offered as a template for your chosen green space, be it your own backyard, another national park, or some other place where you can be in touch with the earth and her creatures. Once again, all that you find there can be available to you throughout life. Gather up the details, create the memories, embed them in your mind, and access them whenever you choose.

So many questions present themselves. When you actively engage in the natural world, what creatures, plants, and geological features might you expect to see? How can these experiences serve as a model for green space engagement, regardless of where you live and travel and regardless of at what stage you are in life? How can you carry with you the memories and the creative imagination to translate these experiences into a treasure trove of visualizations that can last throughout your life? How can you volunteer to assist in ensuring that these places and creatures are healthy and are available in perpetuity? In concert with all of this, how can you care for yourself through healthy exercise, dietary, and support network choices? How can you choose alternative activities that will link you to the natural world during challenging periods?

To work on the answers to these questions, step deeply into these two national parks to discover some of the many opportunities for physical, spiritual, and emotional enrichment that exist there. Much of what you find in the next chapter on Acadia National Park may be familiar to you if you make your home in or travel to any cool climates. Then go to the tropic environment of Virgin Islands National Park that will be more familiar if you are connected to warmer environs.

At times, I will share some personal nature experiences with you as encouragement to delve into more of your own. These tales and the specifics of particular green and blue spaces may help you to build a repertoire of images for your own use. Once again, they serve as a model that you can use to enhance your life as you move into your own chosen spots in the natural world. Build details in your mind of all that is around you, learn and observe all that you can of creatures and places, indulge all of your senses, and carry the memories, real or imagined, on with you throughout your life.

Acadia National Park and its sister park, Virgin Islands National Park, exist primarily on islands in the sea that binds us all together.

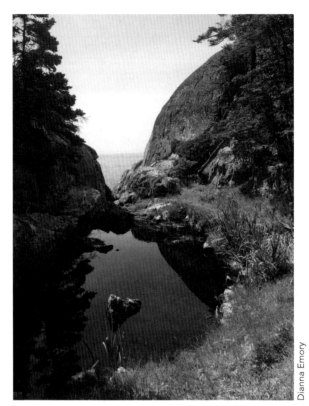

Dianna Emory

Tranquility at Isle au Haut, Acadia National Park.

Through examining much of what these two parks hold, we can use them as templates for thinking about any part of the natural world from our current experience, our memories, or our imaginations. We can tap into these green places and the nearby waters as vehicles to life enrichment. We can use what we find there to positively propel those we love and ourselves through all stages of life and its inevitable challenges. And, we can enrich ourselves with scores of memories and visual images from which we can draw during the times when our ability to get outdoors is limited. I have lived this approach, and I can guarantee that it works.

7

VENTURING FORTH
INTO ACADIA NATIONAL PARK

"All good things are wild and free."
Henry David Thoreau

I hope you have visited Maine's Acadia National Park with its three districts: Mount Desert Island, Isle au Haut, and the Schoodic District, or perhaps the Caribbean island of St. John, home of much of Virgin Islands National Park. If so, you have probably taken away memories and visual images that will serve you well throughout your life. But, even if you are prevented from traveling to these or other magnificent places, learning about their features and their creatures can help you to examine all that is directly around you in more detail. Careful examination can be repeated in many ways to deepen your sensory relationship with the natural world, whether in your immediate surroundings or through broadening your adventures out as far as you are able. We begin with Acadia.

During one of my life valleys, when volunteerism was helping me to hold my life together, I wrote the following column for the *Friends of Acadia Journal*. It illustrates how the natural world—in this case Acadia National Park—can come to one's assistance in many ways.

"The Critical Nature of Green Space"
Reprinted from *Friends of Acadia Journal*, 2004,
Board Chairman's Letter

One year ago, perched on a favorite rocky outcropping, I contemplated the sweeping view and considered how to cope with life's latest challenge. My 34-year-old daughter, Melissa, was in the sixth month of treatment for a very aggressive form of breast cancer. Surgery was behind; another year of chemo, radiation, and an experimental treatment lay ahead. Melissa's active, happy life had been ambushed and there seemed to be no promises for the future. My worst nightmare as a parent had become reality.

The love, support, and prayers that so many of you have offered have been enormously helpful. Thank you. Melissa has successfully completed her first year of treatment and is happily and healthily plunging forward, continuing to give to others while also nurturing herself.

Throughout this ordeal, I have frequently turned to Acadia for support. During the worst of it, the park has welcomed and nurtured me, providing endless opportunities for quiet reflection. Without the runs around the lake, climbs up the West Face, bike rides, and many hours of hiking and cross-country skiing, I would have been missing the glue that has held me together. Many of you have joined me on these expeditions and that has made each one more meaningful.

Most of us have at some point faced a crisis that has demanded that we gather up our resources in order to forge ahead. Green space allows us the opportunity for venting and caring for our bodies through physical activity, time away from the crowds, unobstructed views, and access to beautiful places. With others or alone, we can renew and energize ourselves in a way that is often impossible in the confines of a building or structural intrusion. Time away from the reminders of life's pressures—as well as from the visual and auditory pollution that seems to be ever-present in our society—is critical to our emotional and physical health. During times of stress, these escapes are even more important.

Acadia National Park blesses us with the opportunity for spiritual, physical, and emotional renewal. This column is dedicated to all of you who have found solace in its resources during difficult times and to those who have faced debilitating mental or physical illness. Sometimes even the memories of our times in the park help us to move forward more comfortably. With love and thanks to you all for helping to protect this extraordinary place.

Whenever you need them, the natural world and her creatures are there for you. It is probably easy to see what solace I found in Acadia's offerings during my daughter's treatment and how desolate life might have been for her and for me without access to green spaces. As we examine the details of Acadia and use it as a model for any engagement with the natural world, let's consider how this approach can be used to enhance your own opportunities to connect with the world and her creatures.

BACKGROUND INFORMATION

Acadia National Park's three districts are located on Mount Desert Island (31,000+/- acres), the Schoodic Peninsula (3,500+/- acres), and Isle au Haut (2,730 acres) on the Atlantic Coast of the state of Maine. Conservation easements totaling about 12,000 acres are also held by Acadia on nearly 200 properties, most all of which are on Maine islands. Originally preserved by early 20th century philanthropists, parcels have been added to the Park through 2017. Acadia's rugged granite coastline, forests, and beaches draw over 3 million visitors annually for hiking, biking, equestrian activities, cross-country skiing, sight-seeing, water sports, and interactions with plants and animals.

Primarily a product of marine influences and latitude, Acadia's climate ranges from 90 degree summer days to winter temperatures below zero, according to the Park. In general, temperatures are more moderate and snowfall is less than inland Maine. Average annual rainfall is four feet while average annual snowfall is five feet.

Acadia National Park is assisted in its efforts by Friends of Acadia, Schoodic Institute at Acadia National Park, Maine Coast Heritage Trust, Mount Desert Biological Laboratory, College of the Atlantic, and other conservation partners.

In the interest of cleaner air and less traffic, all Acadia parking lots and many other points can be easily accessed through the Island Explorer, a fare-free propane-powered bus system. Through a partnership with Friends of Acadia, since 2002 LL Bean has contributed more than $3.5 million to help to protect Acadia National Park through supporting scientific research, youth programs, and the bus system. As Janet Wyper, Manager of Community Relations of LL Bean, stated in 2016, "It is a natural fit for our company to sponsor the Island Explorer, which has enabled millions of people to enjoy one of Maine's and the nation's greatest natural assets, Acadia National Park, in an

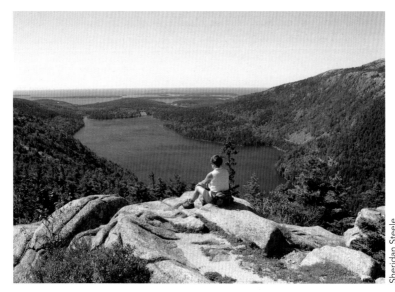

Sheridan Steele

Contemplating Nature from South Bubble, Acadia National Park.

environmentally-friendly manner." During the early years of the Island Explorer, it was my pleasure to work closely with former Friends of Acadia president, Ken Olson, and members of the LL Bean leadership team, including Chris McCormick, Janet Wyper, Stafford Soule, and others. The Bean team went beyond sending a positive conservation message and making financial contributions when they sent a large group of employees to help groom and rake the carriage roads of Acadia, one more labor of love from people who treasure the natural world.

THE LANDS OF ACADIA NATIONAL PARK

Do you have a favorite activity that transports you to a state where your body and your mind can be restored? Are there places that you know so well that you can conjure up specifics related to their sights, sounds, smells, and tastes just by thinking about them? Using Acadia as a model, begin to create as much detail as you can about those places and the creatures you find there as you engage in your chosen activities.

As we delve into Acadia, please note that the more detail you find, the more material you will have for the times when you are on overload or are slowed down physically and can't get outdoors as much as you want. Acadia and Virgin Islands National Park are models with which I happen to be very familiar. You can apply all that is available there to your own green space, wherever you may be.

What are the activities you gravitate toward during each season? You might want to list them and think about how they fit with what Acadia offers. Then, as we look at the details of adventures in Acadia, create a sensory memory of your adventures in places that you cherish. Record or etch in your mind details of specific expeditions.

Acadia in the winter presents 45 miles of carriage roads for cross-country skiing; winter hiking and climbing on more than 125 miles of trails; ice skating on 26 ponds and lakes; and icy rowing, paddle boarding, sea kayaking, and frost-bite sailing on the ocean that surrounds the Mount Desert Island District of Acadia National Park. The Park's Schoodic and Isle au Haut Districts provide similar experiences, but are wilder than MDI.

Spring, summer, and fall offer endless runs, hikes, bike rides, climbs, and horseback adventures over the mountains, through the Park's valleys, and along the shoreline. Fresh and salt waters promise invigorating stand-up paddle boarding, canoeing, rowing, kayaking, sailing, swimming, and cool-water snorkeling/diving. No motors are permitted on the carriage roads or trails of Acadia except for two locations near Eagle Lake and Jordan Pond. The paved Park Loop Road allows snowmobiling in winter.

A look at specific areas for these activities is offered in a number of guidebooks and on the websites of Acadia National Park, Friends of Acadia, Schoodic Institute at Acadia National Park, Maine Coast Heritage Trust, Maine Island Trail Association, and other organizations. I hope you will also enjoy some of my favorite expeditions, as their descriptions provide fodder for your own visualization scripts. As a very active athlete nearing seven decades, I am also rating some activities according to two levels of difficulty. Start with the level that feels comfortable to you for each activity and build up to something more. And remember, even if you are slowed down or brought to a screeching halt, you will likely return to your former level of activity after the crisis. If not, there are so many other ways to experience the green spaces that you love. I am reminded of a recent *New York Times* column that relates the feelings of novelist and nature and travel writer Edward Hoagland, who went blind several years ago. As Jane Brody writes, "Of course, he sorely misses nature's inspiring vistas and inhabitants that fueled his writing, though he can still hear birds chatter in the trees, leaves rustle in the wind and waves crash on the shore."[42]

As we take a look at the outdoor activities available to those who enjoy Acadia National Park, you will read about special places and activities that have made memories and presented a wealth of material for creating visualizations. If you don't find your way to Acadia, please use it as a model for any green space that you can access.

Potential expeditions cover miles of stunning trails and carriage roads, described in detail in Tom St. Germain's *A Walk in the Park.*[43] Dolores Kong and Dan Ring are co-authors of two Falcon guides, *Hiking Acadia National Park*[44] and *Best Easy Day Hikes, Acadia National Park.*[45] Their blog, acadiaonmymind.com, provides a wealth of information related to flora, fauna, advocacy issues, and threats to Acadia National Park. Trekking along the trails of Isle au Haut one summer day, immersed in conversation about threats to Acadia's natural resources, we scrambled down a cliff face and around a corner to find Dolores and Dan discussing other Acadia issues. Ambassadors like the Kong-Rings do much for the natural world. You can join them by volunteering for Friends of Acadia, Maine Coast Heritage Trust, Schoodic Institute, or an organization near you.

For the fun of it, I am sharing a few of the routes that I love running, skiing, or hiking. Anything you explore in all districts of Acadia, will be a thrill you will not forget. You will find a host of lovely vistas, exquisite plants and trees, gorgeous water features, abundant wildlife, and many hours of workouts for your mind and your body. The wealth of memories and visual images you collect will last you for the rest of your life.

Hiking and Running Acadia

Hiking and running over the carriage roads and trails of Acadia National Park are an athlete's dream. An added pleasure is riding your bike to a trailhead, doing a run/hike, and then rejoining your bike for more carriage road riding. It is an absolute joy to pack water and food and head off into this park where you will encounter no worrisome plants or wildlife, other than deer ticks and the occasional poison ivy. Tuck long pants into your socks and spray with DEET to discourage ticks. Shower and wash clothing in hot water as soon as you get home.

The following sections, plus the Appendix to Chapter Seven, found on my website, hold samples of favorite hiking, skiing, and running expeditions.

Favorite Hikes and Runs
More Challenging Hiking and Running:

Mount Desert District: Lower Hadlock parking lot to lower portion of Hadlock Loop, to Amphitheater upper carriage road, to connector carriage road to Penobscot Mountain trail. Up Penobscot trail to Penobscot summit, return to carriage road via Spring Trail. Return to parking lot via Amphitheater and lower Hadlock Loop.

Mount Desert District: Bubble Pond parking lot up the West Face of Cadillac Mountain, down the South Ridge to the Featherbed and the intersection with the Cannon Brook Trail, down the old Pond Trail to the Bubble Pond carriage road, follow Bubble Pond shore back to parking lot.

Mount Desert District: Upper Parkman parking lot up the Hadlock Loop, up Parkman Mountain carriage road, up Parkman Mountain trail to summit, down Parkman trail to carriage road, down Parkman carriage road to intersect Hadlock Loop, around remainder of Hadlock Loop back to car.

Mount Desert District: Champlain Mountain from Route 3 parking lot to The Bowl and back, or leave one car to depart from Sand Beach area to climb The Beehive up Champlain, ending at Route 3 and a second car.

Isle au Haut District: Duck Harbor Landing up Duck Harbor Mountain, down Duck Harbor Mountain Trail to the Goat Trail, following the Goat Trail to the Island Loop Road, which you follow until you see the short trail back to Duck Harbor Landing.

Schoodic District: All Schoodic Woods gravel roads and trails. Wow! Thank you to the donors of this most recent addition to Acadia National Park.

Easy Hiking, Running, and Skiing:
Mount Desert District of Acadia National Park:
> Hadlock Loop
> Eagle Lake Loop
> Witch Hole Pond Loop (Paradise Hill Loop can be combined
with this.)
> Little Long Pond Loop
> Amphitheater Loop, accessed via Lower Hadlock carriage road.
> Dorr Mountain

Isle au District of Acadia National Park:
> Duck Harbor walk to town

Schoodic District of Acadia National Park:
> Campus of Schoodic Institute at Acadia National Park and
Schoodic Point
> Lower sections of Schoodic Woods network

Cross-Country Skiing and Ice Skating Acadia

Do you have an activity that provides a relationship for you as it transports you to a better place? Skiing Acadia is the winter sport of my soul. Gliding gracefully along the carriage roads on perfectly waxed skis is a thrilling thing that can be easily recalled even on a summer day.

This day, however, begins at 17 degrees, requiring layers of extra clothing and toe-warming packets, but the soft, deep powder is so inviting. Years ago, we broke our own trails and skied all day up, down, and around Acadia's mountains. Now, volunteer track-setters, using equipment purchased by Friends of Acadia, spend endless hours—often in the middle of the night—preparing perfect conditions for Nordic and skate skiing. Today I start at the Visitor's Center, follow the Witch Hole Pond carriage road to Eagle Lake, head off to Aunt Betty's Pond, up the Seven Bridges, back along the east side of Eagle Lake, and over to and around the remainder of the Witch Hole Pond Trail. En route, I encounter Acadia's Park Superintendent, Kevin Schneider, skiing happily along enjoying this place that he leads and protects so capably. "Did you see those fox tracks heading across the pond?" I ask. "I started to follow the tracks and they just ended. Then I stuck my head in the culvert and found a fox home!" Do not stick your head into just any old hole, or you might just find a porcupine butt.

For many years, my skis felt like another set of appendages, offering headlamp-lit early morning solitary expeditions, lengthy picnic skis with friends and family, and a convincing reason to spend time in this winter place with its short days and frigid temperatures. One magical night, Ben and I skied to Witch Hole Pond under a full moon. Out on the pond, we marveled at the Hale Bopp Comet, the moon, the stars, and the mountains of Acadia etched against the sky. The bliss of flying down the Sargent Mountain carriage road inhaling the brisk Maine air is another Acadian adventure you will not forget. Just breathe in deeply now and imagine…

While it is not available as frequently as the skiing, there is nothing finer than shooting on ice skates up Northeast Creek amidst the frozen cranberries, into the side streams and wetlands, investigating haunts of eagles, ducks, muskrats, beaver, and deer. On a day when there is snow on the ground but the ponds are bare—a rare thing, ski into Aunt Betty's Pond, Witch Hole Pond, or the Bubbles to find yourselves alone in the Park, with nature surrounding you. Each time we skate Aunt Betty's, memories flood in of times with my friends, Clare and Helen, who left this world too soon. Their spirits join me there, laughing as we fly around and around the pond, all rosy-cheeked and fit. Do you have special places that remind you of others? Let's pause for a moment and go to one of those places right now through your mind's eye. What memories come back to you of times shared there with a treasured person? How does that place in nature help you to hold on to someone who is no longer in this world? How blessed are some places in this world for their ability to bring loved ones lost back into our thoughts. Sometimes, it almost feels like they are there beside us, doesn't it?

Biking Acadia

The 27-mile Park Loop Road is a magnificent blend of ocean views, bold mountain cliffs, quiet ponds, bird-watching, and wildlife encounters. It is a pleasure to bike the Loop during mud season when Acadia's carriage roads are closed until they are dry enough not to incur damage from feet, hooves, or bikes. On this particular day, as we pump up hills and speed down their back sides, there is the anticipation of the remains of a night of sixty knot winds. We are not disappointed. At every ocean sighting, huge rollers sweep toward ledges and cliffs with foam and surf shooting high into the sky. From our bikes, we note the unusual color of the sea, much more the aqua of tropic waters due, perhaps, to the mist-filled air and the strength of the waves on the shallow bottom. Once from this view overlooking Frenchman Bay, Ironbound Island, and Egg Rock, we were astounded to gaze down on a large whale swimming slowly just beneath the ocean's surface. Later that day, we reported the sighting to Dr. Steve Katona, one of the world's leading marine mammal experts and a former president of College of the Atlantic. Steve said, smiling knowingly, "They are there. You were in the right place at the right time."

Another day on this loop, Bear Brook Pond shines ahead with what look like little brown things floating around. As I get closer, I notice one moving. An otter! Make that five. Wow! Two adults and three yearling otters! We return on other spring days and find them more and more curious, swimming close along the shore for mutual inspection.

If you love biking, you will love what awaits you on the carriage roads. Due to their gravel base, they are not easy for road bikes, but hybrid and mountain bikers can travel speedily along while observing the Rules of the Road. There is nothing so uplifting as several hours biking in the Mount Desert District of Acadia and now on the new bike trails at Schoodic Woods in the Schoodic District. Isle au Haut has its bumps, but that is fun as well. You can surely create more memories in each district.

All carriage roads and the Park Loop Road are bike-friendly, but no bikes are permitted on the trail network. For the fun of it, I will share some of my favorites with you, although I will leave the guidebooks to the professionals.

Favorite Bike Rides

From ANP Visitors' Center, up access trail to Witch Hole Loop, right around Loop to connector to Eagle Lake carriage road, up Aunt Betty's Pond carriage road after bridge, past Aunt Betty's Pond, up Seven Bridges, up Sargent Mountain carriage road, down Sargent Mountain carriage road to Hadlock Loop, right and down Hadlock Loop, connecting to Brown Mountain carriage road, Brown Mountain carriage road back to Aunt Betty's Pond Marsh, left and up Aunt Betty's carriage road below ANP Headquarters, down to connect with Eagle Lake carriage road to connector to Witch Hole Pond carriage road, left on Witch Hole Pond carriage road back to access trail to Visitor's Center parking lot.

From Schoodic Woods Visitor's Center, Schoodic District, Acadia National Park, pick up a trail map and head off to explore every inch of these marvelous trails, recently created by generous philanthropists who donated the Center and its lands to Acadia.

From Schoodic Education and Research Center/Schoodic Institute at Acadia National Park bike around the campus to explore all that it holds. Do the quick dead end ride to Schoodic Point, then head off to bike the entire Park paved road and part of the main road to make a big loop. Side trips into the Schoodic Woods area will provide additional great biking.

Ferry from Stonington to Isle au Haut District, Acadia National Park, off-load at Duck Harbor landing or town dock (Duck Harbor landing is seasonal). Rough gravel roads traverse the island and the Park, providing fun, but bumpy, biking.

Horses in Acadia

Before the days of large bike tour groups, whose riders seem to have little knowledge of horse etiquette, we cantered confidently along the carriage roads. The children took off on their own and learned about the Park from the backs of their horses. Sometimes, the horses were the guides, as on the day when several of us trotted around the Amphitheater and I looked behind me to check on four-year-old Bethany. No Bethany. No Blaze. A quick canter back to a side trail and a trot through the woods found Bethany and Blaze lumbering back in my direction.

There was a time when the carriage roads were in poor condition. Galloping around the Amphitheatre another summer day, my horse plunged one leg through the road as I flew through the air to slam my head into a coping stone. Miraculously, Chiclet suffered no injuries. I, on the other hand, headed off the next day to present a keynote conference speech with a concussion and many scrapes. Another afternoon, we trotted across a wooden bridge and went through that as well. Now, those accidents would not occur, thanks to constant maintenance work in the Park. These tales reinforce the great importance of the Acadia National Park staff, Friends of Acadia, and the many philanthropists who have contributed to the restoration of the carriage roads and trail systems. Others donate hours rebuilding bridges, clearing vistas, and cleaning ditches. In Chapter Ten, we will get to the importance of

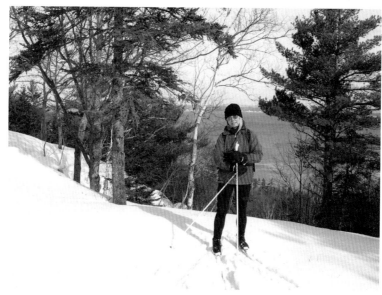

Ben Emory

Winter Bliss on Parkman Mountain, Acadia National Park.

volunteerism and the many ways you can engage in your own community to really make a difference—to yourself and to the world that you steward.

All roads of Isle au Haut and all carriage roads of the Mount Desert District, except the Witch Hole Pond carriage road and a portion of the Eagle Lake carriage road, are horse-friendly. No horses are permitted on the trail network.

THE WATERS AROUND ACADIA NATIONAL PARK

"The notion that the ocean that I grew up with is not something that I can pass on to my kids is unacceptable." President Barack Obama at the designation of the Canyons National Monument, 2016.

Bodies of water, fresh and salt, offer us another way to explore the natural world. Regardless of the craft, from kayak to paddle boarding to rowboat to sailing vessel, adventures upon the waters hold universal appeal, offering us the opportunity to be away from the hurly burly. We can traverse the marshlands watching for birds, head across a lake toward the setting sun, run the river rapids in a kayak, or climb aboard a boat in Maine and sail across the seas to other lands and new adventures. A sense of freedom and the chance to put one's life in perspective ensues. Regardless of where you are, there is likely a pond, river, lake, or ocean within driving distance. The opportunities for water-based recreation and connections to nature await you. As you engage with the fresh and salt waters, follow the same procedure that you did when we focused on the land. Record the experiences in your mind, write about and connect with the details of all that you see, touch, taste, smell, and hear, and practice recalling the minutiae. Here are some examples of what you can find in Acadia and how to recall experiences there.

Stand-up Paddle Boarding (SUPing), Rowing, Kayaking, and Canoeing Acadia National Park

(All paddle boarding expeditions could be done by rowboat or kayak. Safer canoeing exists on lakes and ponds.)

Popping out at dawn through their boat's companionway, Beth and Don Straus beckon to us. Anchored not far away, we watch their white heads as they climb down into their rowboat and Don hollers, "You've never seen us row together. Wait until you see this!" We watch in awe as they stroke perfectly in tandem, the bow of their dinghy cutting smoothly through the dark Maine waters. They spin and come up alongside our boat, clambering aboard. We compliment their rowing elegance, and Beth replies, "No matter how you start your day, by the time you return from a row, everything is in perfect harmony." Until our son, Thor, gave us the paddle boarding bug, we double-rowed year-round every day that we could haul a boat through the ice or challenge the wind. I suspect that when we age-out of paddle boarding, we will go back to the double-rowing, a sport that one can enjoy for nearly a lifetime and which will take you to magical places. Rowers or not, start your day doing something you love with a special person and, as Beth said, "Everything will be in perfect harmony."

Crunching with my step, the frozen seaweed promises ice on Frenchman Bay for this paddle boarding addict. The mercury bumps 32 degrees, but a dry suit, mittens, two hats, and a life jacket guarantee a purging sweat. Gliding smoothly through the glassy water, the sudden tinkle of skim ice shattering reminds me of the cautions of winter paddle board-ing. When skim ice is too thick, it can bring the board to a screeching halt with the threat of a frigid plunge. Those are days to choose a differ-ent sport. But today, the ice is melting as I paddle hard along the shore, over ledges sharing glimpses of the entrancing world that lives around them. Rockweed floats toward the surface, calling out the critical nature of this ocean alga and the host of creatures that it serves. On summer days, a snorkeling expedition pawing through the rockweed looking for crabs, tiny fish, and other creatures draws one into an environment des-perately begging for protection. Today, I round the corner toward The Ovens, a fascinating series of oceanside caves, which today are decorated by huge stalactite-like icicles. Looking down through 15 feet of crystal waters, I see many hundreds of black sand dollars scattered over this sandy portion of the ocean floor. I have never seen so many and assume that this particular bottom draws them for reproduction.

It is November, a flat-air overcast day of 49 degrees in eastern Maine. The snapdragons still kick out a few blossoms and moths flit across the night sky as I prepare to head off across the bay with no fear of cold hands or feet. It is unsettling to look back at this warm fall, considering that we often have had several snows and many hard freezes by now. While I am pulling on my booties, *The New York Times* on the counter showcases its article on the threat of rising sea level to coastal real estate. Many climate change deniers are going to find their homes at risk, but some seem to find solace in the fact that insurance will always replace the structures. I shake my head, trying to clear it of the threat to the environment feared by our like-minded peers. Through volunteer efforts and contributions of time, energy, and dollars, we do what we can. We feel rewarded for that in the multitude of outdoor adventures that await us at every turn. But, we also tear up and worry at the thought of what the future might—or might not—hold for our children and grandchildren. For now, I race down the hill to our gravel beach, slip my paddle board into the water, and zip toward Ben who is climbing into our rowboat. In the breaking dawn, we head across the bay, with its views of Mount Desert Island and the Schoodic Peninsula's Acadia National Park playgrounds. Thousands work to protect this mecca of recreation and relaxation on behalf of its natural resources and over 3.2 million visitors who make their way to this spectacular park each summer.

On paddle boards, we have closely explored the best of Maine's coastal destinations, discovering shallow water jewels. We have added another dimension to an intimate connection with this magnificent coast. Thrilled to paddle above all else, I have restricted my long distance running to days when there is a gale or a blizzard. And, when I planted my leg through a Virgin Gorda cattle guard and fell at a 90-degree angle, much of the recovery of my shattered limb was thanks to the therapeutic benefit of stand-up paddle boarding.

Paddle boarding-related wildlife encounters enhance each venture, making the trip much more than a health-benefiting, athletic expedition. As my board scoots along, a whiskery snout pokes from the dark waters off Chatto Island, followed by a horsehead seal's bulbous cow eyes. A rarity in Brooklin's Center Harbor, she follows me across Eggemoggin Reach on this fine summer day, diving and splashing in the grandeur of her island-studded home, passing several of her harbor seal cousins along the way. The smooth, undulating surface of the Reach reflects the rosy dawn, inviting my skimming across its surface. Three mackerel-feeding porpoises rise and fall in unison—likely the same playful gang I see regularly. One morning brought them streaming along to cross my wake and dive close under my board; another saw me joining them to swim as they dove and splashed around.

A loon calls out and terns flit by as I approach the Eastern Torrey Island shore, while my seal friend snorts, humps her back, and plummets down to head back across the Reach. As I paddle along, my vantage point allows close examination of the weed below, with occasional glimpses of tiny silvery fish. I don my snorkel and mask, stick my head over the bow, and paw my way through deep-rooted clumps of rockweed, then over eelgrass. As I peer through my mask, the slippery eelgrass looks healthier and more expansive than it did a year ago. Tiny hermit crabs inhabiting periwinkle shells skitter along, beckoning me to stay, but I stand and paddle rapidly along the Torrey shores, through the Gap, and on toward Babson Island as the breeze begins to build.

Cutting across the Reach, my bow takes frequent waves as I paddle harder, contemplating what lies below the surface, while absorbing the multitude of island nooks and crannies ripe for exploration. The scent of the sea and bait is strong as lobster boats arrive to churn the waters while traps are hauled. Big wakes from several directions combine with the building sea to create a confused surface chop across the Reach. Paddling hard upwind while navigating the chop and wakes requires attention, but my mind and body still absorb the overwhelming beauty of sky and sea and shore. In the distance, Acadia's Isle au Haut District beckons, as does Maine Coast Heritage Trust's magnificent Marshall Island. Reassurance comes in the fact that so many of these islands are

protected, thanks to the generosity of their owners and the effectiveness of Maine Coast Heritage Trust, Acadia National Park, and other
conservation-related entities. What a gift this is to paddle boarders,
kayakers, island explorers, and boaters of all sorts. Spanning the Reach,
I see MCHT's Hog and Bear, and seven of the islands on which Acadia holds conservation easements. Privately owned, this group includes
forever-wild Chatto Island, which protects Center Harbor. Paddling
near the Chatto shore one day brought an encounter with three river
otters, residents of this protected island gem.

   With Chatto in my sight, I turn and fly downwind across the
Reach, over the Chatto bar, up and around the shallow head of Center
Harbor, through the fleet near Brooklin Boat Yard, and back to our
dock and family. Like my bike, my running legs, my skis, our boats, and
my horses past, this board recharges me, gives me one more touchstone
with the natural world, and keeps my body and soul fit and happy.

A brisk wind takes us from Mount Desert to Acadia's Schoodic District,
past Petit Manan National Wildlife Refuge and on east of Acadia where
Washington County holds a host of captivating coves less travelled, ripe
for exploration by boat, SUP, rowing vessel, or kayak. The Roque Island
archipelago, from Roque's sweeping Great Beach up the Thoroughfare
to Great Spruce Island's Bunker Cove, is a five-star expedition. On a
calm day, the Great Beach offers a lovely anchorage where the generous
owners permit walking along the eastern end of the beach. Enticing
stand-up paddle boarding, rowing, or kayaking abounds, whether skirting along the shore, up into Lakeman's or choosing a stiff paddle in a
strong current through the Thoroughfare. But, the best is yet to come.
Rounding the corner into Bunker Cove, along both shores are a myriad
of coves and a split into the open ocean.

   This September day, we are protected from strong ocean swells
as we paddle into side coves, examining shoreline, birds, and vegetation. Kingfishers abound, their chatter echoing as they zoom across the
cove. A break in the cove offers open ocean views, where swells crash

in upon the granite shore. Reef-like ledges admit big rollers, inviting us to paddle upwind to turn and ride the roll across the cove. Two harbor seals follow close behind us, poking long snouts and big cow eyes in our direction. A lone eagle soars as pipers flit along the shore.

Our eyes squint at three tawny lumps basking on sunshine-warmed granite. Hard to see, but they look like the coyotes we saw one winter day across Frost Pond. We like thinking of them here, unthreatened in the sun, unlike our Frost Pond coyotes whom bounty hunters took away.

This group could just be rocks, but we will call them coyotes while we paddle deeper into Bunker Cove. The Cove's head offers panoramic views of this remarkable downeast jewel where a sheer 60-foot drop from one bold ledge stands out along the eastern shore. We paddle close, ducking under mountain ash laden with fat red berries, food for the birds' taking. Every corner promises a resolution to the coyote question. We round each one, expecting three tubular brown boulders, not the hoped-for coyotes. We are reminded of a crisp fall day when we rowed our peapod into the deepest cove here to spot a great horned owl perched upon a dead tree branch. Surveying us carefully as he swung his head around, he blinked large eyes, raised his wings, and disappeared into the thick spruce forest. Entering this cove always holds the hope of another owl sighting. Today we are thinking about coyotes, as well as owls.

Soon the corner to the Thoroughfare appears. We have found no trio of tawny boulders along the shore. Hopefully, we think, three coyotes might have basked on a sun-drenched shore, restoring paddlers' dreams of coyotes free.

Now it is your turn again. If you are headed for Maine, try to choose at least three locations there, learn everything you can about them, and go there. Whatever your favorite location, list three places that you especially enjoy. Learn everything you can about them. List two of your favorite activities that you can engage in while visiting those places. Put in as much detail as you can about the places, the activities, and the sensory experiences that they hold.

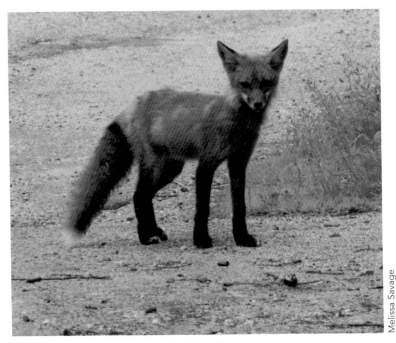

Red Fox Kit.

FAUNA OF ACADIA NATIONAL PARK
Creatures of the Lands of Acadia National Park

Many wild creatures frequent the Acadia region. You may know these animals. Perhaps some of them are in your own backyard! An early morning walk to Witch Hole Pond can bring the mesmerizing experience of watching beavers chop down trees three times bigger around than their furry bottoms and haul them to their lodges; ducks with tails in the air and heads under water as they scoop up breakfast; or resident otters playfully sliding down the rocks into the pond below. In winter, the same otters pop their heads up through ice-fishing holes to surprise skaters and fishermen.

Evening expeditions bring out the owls, the little brown bats, peeper frogs, and more of the Park's deer herd. White-tailed deer abound in Acadia. Lovely, graceful creatures, they and their fawns gallop across our fields, playing tag with one another. One can sometimes even catch a glimpse of an albino deer that frequents the Park and has become quite accustomed to humans. An important deer-related note is that outdoorspeople must be cognizant of Lyme disease and other ailments carried by the ticks harbored by deer and other mammals. DEET repellent, daily tick checks, hot showers, and immediate hot washing and drying of clothing are preventative approaches. Infectious disease expert Dr. Peter Rand announced one day, when I rejoiced that winter provided me the opportunity to scramble though the bushes without worry of ticks, "The next time you go bushwacking in the snow, drag a piece of white flannel behind you." I did. Yuck. It was covered with ticks. Be vigilant, but march out the door and enjoy yourself.

There are foxes and minks, mice and voles, chipmunks and squirrels, bobcats and ermine, the occasional bear or moose, and numerous packs of very healthy German shepherd-sized coyotes. The coyotes tend to stand their ground—intimidating behavior—waiting for you to skirt around them or haul your bike up over the hillside.

You might want to focus on a few of these animals and learn everything you can about them. Study their appearance and their behavior and etch the memory of their form, scent, voice, and tracks in your mind. Following are some of the wildlife I have seen in Acadia. For more, please go to the Appendix for Chapter Seven on my website. Whether you choose to focus on the ones for which I have shared tales or on some of the others, you are encouraged to pick at least one creature from each category and study it in detail. It is terrific if you can see the real animal. If not, find out all that you can about them and study their photos so that you can later build them into a visualization exercise. For a few, you might write a paragraph about an encounter from your memory or your imagination and some of the thoughts stimulated by that experience. For a brain-stimulating adventure, memorize the Latin names.

Animals Sighted in Acadia National Park

REPTILES (partial list)
TURTLES
Painted Turtle (*Chrysemys picta*)

Today I saved a painted turtle. He sat mid-road between the two ponds, apparently undecided as to which pond might hold more allure and oblivious to a whizzing car's potential to shatter his life. Parking in the soft shoulder, but careful to avoid the areas where his bigger snapper cousins had nested, I hopped down from my Jeep and approached the little hump on the pavement. Had he already been hit and wounded, or worse? I carefully picked up the softball-sized little guy, prepared to find his shell cracked, with a limp head and legs dangling out. Head and appendages shot out of the shell and sharp little toenails clawed the air frantically, attempting to find some solid ground. I carried the very-much-alive turtle to the bank of his apparent destination, placed him carefully on the edge of the lily-filled pond, and watched him scramble into the water. Soon, his small dark head poked above the surface and the sunlight kissed his tiny nose. He looked around, ducked under, and was gone.

In my next life I may be a herpetologist, studying and protecting these creatures. Melissa and I share this fascination with turtles—she going so far as to have an Amsterdam tattoo artist create a reptilian image on her arm. What began as a small turtle grew with the artist's creativity. Unwilling to insult the artist or hurt his feelings, Liss allowed him to continue in his craft as the turtle grew to fill a large portion of her upper arm. Upon her return from the semester in Holland, a horrified mother was not as enamored with the turtle art as its wearer. In later years, the turtle tattoo seems to have become a protective and friendly symbol to Melissa. Turtle tattoos, prayers, friends, family, doctors, chemo, radiation, surgery, whatever it takes. Please let all of this be enough to protect her from this illness. If only I could pick Melissa up, lift her out of harm's way and carry her to safety as easily as I moved that painted turtle and gave him another chance at life.

Snapping Turtle (*Chelydra serpentina*)
Returning from a blueberrying expedition with my beloved Nanny, we drew closer and closer to a large black hump on the roadside. We stopped short, in respect for the huge snapper, and my adventurous grandmother held out a hefty stick. "Snap," went the completely severed stick.

SNAKES

All of the following snakes were found when they were much thinner and much shorter than a pencil. As a child captivated by all living things, I was delighted to raise them in my terrariums. My ever-tolerant parents rarely complained until the snakes began to escape their homes.

Common Garter Snake (*Thamnophis sirtalis*)

Milk Snake/Spotted Adder (*Lampropeltis triangulum triangulum*)

Northern Red-bellied Snake (*Storeria occipitomaculata occipitomaculata*)

Northern Ringneck Snake (*Diadophis punctatus edwardsi*)

Smooth Green Snake (*Liochlorophis vernalis*)

AMPHIBIANS (partial list)

University of Maine professors Alan O'Connell, Malcolm Hunter, William Glanz, and Aram Calhoun report that fourteen species of amphibians have been recorded on Mount Desert Island.

FROGS AND TOADS

American Toad (*Bufo americanus*)
Gardeners are thrilled to find a toad amidst the foliage, as something about them says, "Good luck." Devourers of insects, they help to naturally protect our plants from chewing creatures.

Bullfrog (*Rana catesbeiana*)
Close in appearance to the green frog, the bullfrog holds the title of "largest frog." Bullfrogs have yellow bellies, while green frogs sport whiter bellies.

Gray Treefrog (*Hyla versicolor*)
With great excitement, my young garden helper calls me to the daylilies
and reports, "The fairy frogs are here!" Deep within the throats of many
daylilies, tiny sticky-footed frogs peek out. Never again will I look at
a daylily without trying to see a fairy frog within. Sometimes they are
there.

Green Frog (*Rana clamitans*)
One of the two largest frogs, green frogs can be identified by the ridges
that extend from behind their eyes down their backs.

Leopard Frog (*Rana pipiens*)
Driving along, my mind drifts to nonprofit fundraising projects as the
corner of my eye catches movement at the far right of my field of vision.
Slowing a bit, I am bug-eyed at the sight of a leopard frog hopping
across my dashboard. I pull to the side of the road; take a photo; put
my open palm on the dashboard; he hops in; and I transport him to
the roadside ditch. The natural world will find you no matter where
you are.

Pickerel Frog (*Rana palustris*)
Similar to the leopard frog, the only way to differentiate the two is that
the leopard frog's spots are rounder.

Spring Peeper (*Pseudacris crucifer*)
How many spring peepers must there be to produce the intensity of
sound we hear in marshlands? Harbingers of early spring, their chorus
lulls us to sleep as we ponder the thousands of little creatures filling the
marsh at Meadow Brook with their song. These tiny frogs are marked
by an X on their back.

SALAMANDERS AND NEWTS (partial list)

Eastern Newt (*Notophthalmus viridescens*)
Since discovering a healthy eastern newt population in a eutrophying
pond several years ago, we have returned each spring to watch them.
Last year, they vanished along with the abundant pollywog population.
This spring, they did not return. Where did they go and why? Has
eutrophication reached the point that oxygen is too scarce for their

survival? Off to the web I go to learn the answer. We could learn something about every creature on these lists on the web and see their photos, too. What potential there is for our elder years!

Red-backed Salamander (*Plethodon cinereus*)
Hours of my youth were spent searching under logs, rocks, and leaves for redbacks, some of my favorite companions. They crawled up my arms and over my head and came home to live in my terrariums. Now, when I find them, they remain in their home, where they signal a healthy woodland.

Spotted Salamander (*Ambystoma maculatum*)
The thrill of finding a spotted salamander remains with me. These large, plump salamanders with their yellow spots are wonderful pets, but they are even better in their woodland or garden homes where they devour slugs, snails, and insects. Spotted salamanders are one of many reasons I do not use pesticides, herbicides, or other poisons.

Northern Dusky Salamander (*Desmognathus fuscus*) is of the lungless salamander family.

Four-toed Salamander (*Hemidactylium scutatum)* has four toes on his hind feet.

Northern Two-lined Salamander (*Eurycea bislineata*) is often found in water, including puddles. While the redbacks lived in my terrariums as a child, the Northern two-lined fellows lived in the aquariums.[83]

MAMMALS (partial list)

Bear, Black (*Ursus americanus*)
"Don't turn around fast, but turn around. There is a bear behind you," I say to Ben as we chew our oatmeal and a large black bear strolls past the window of our farmhouse. We have put conservation easements on this property to protect the many creatures that roam its fields and hillsides, the nesting birds, and the rare plants. A bear visit is a wonderful treat. Did you know they can gallop? "Oh, my God, a black cow," I shout to Melissa as we run across the blueberry barrens. Ahead is a large, black galloping animal. "MOM, that is a BEAR!" We watch,

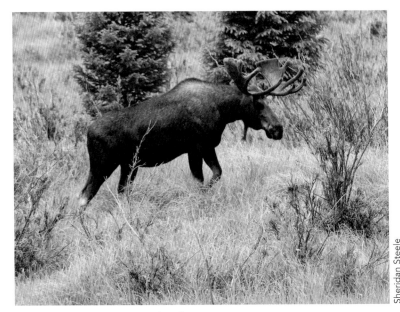

Sheridan Steele

The Elusive Moose.

awestruck, as the lovely beast heads for the woods, long black hair glistening in the sun.

Beaver (*Castor canadensis*)
The ground is crisp and frozen, the grasses covered with frost, as we shiver in the early spring dawn. Flat on our bellies, Julie and I await movement. Like clockwork, the beavers appear, gliding across the still surface of Witch Hole Pond. This is our reward for rising early. Birds stir, singing morning songs, as otter heads appear—one, two, three—bringing more delight than ever expected.

Fox, Eastern Red (*Vulpes vulpes*)
Little fox foot imprints cross the pristine snow of the Witch Hole marsh, ending abruptly at the carriage road. No tracks appear on the other side. Sticking my head inside the carriage road culvert, I find a cozy fox home.

Moose (*Alces alces*)

It is an embarrassing thing to admit that, despite reaching my senior years as an outdoor addict in Maine, I have never seen a moose in the wild. Wyoming? Yes. Newfoundland? Yes. Maine? Everyone I know has seen multiple moose, and they have been on our property numerous times. I have seen their tracks. My friend, Julie, even saw a moose swimming across Somes Sound, and we had three at once in our field. Ben saw them. I remain moose-less.

Mouse, White-Footed (*Peromyscus leucopus*)

No old house is complete without a mouse or two on occasion. The downside is that the white-footed mouse is a prime carrier of the deer tick that is responsible for several tick-borne diseases, including Lyme disease.

Otter (*Lontra canadensis*)

Two smooth otter trails glide down through the forested hillside, stopping abruptly at the pond's edge. Far across the glistening surface of the snow-covered pond, up pop the otters through a well-maintained hole.

Porcupine (*Erethivon dorsatum*)

Have you ever seen a porcupine village? Some day when snow covers the ground, look for a dirty track covered in sawdust. Follow that track to a cave of roots or a woodpile. As you peer inside, you may be so fortunate as to see a fat, quilled butt sticking out. That would be your porcupine who, after a busy day of chewing trees, has dragged himself though the sawdust at the base of his tree and slogged his way through the snow all the way back to his home. On one cross-country ski adventure, Ben and I found eight porcupines ensconced in eight homes in a porcupine village.

Raccoon (*Procyon lotor*)

At age ten, in the days when they were still acceptable pets, I had a pet raccoon named Cuddles. Cuddles arrived nestled in our neighbor's palm, with his eyes still closed. For many days, we fed him through an eye dropper as he gained strength and size. He box-trained and had free run of our cottage until my parents decided it was time for a nice cage. Over the summer he grew and changed, as did my sister and I.

He joined us on walks on his leash and moved with us to Camp Wawenock, across the cove, where he was a special friend to all. In the fall, Cuddles was allowed to run free. Each of us harbored a secret fear that the winter would be the end of him, but he returned to our cottage door each summer shortly after we arrived. Soon, a number of raccoons were in close residence. Over the years, all were called Cuddles.

Weasel, Short-tailed/Ermine (*Mustela erminea*)
Weasels, brown in summer, become the beautiful white ermines that blend so nicely into the snow. Renowned for eating chickens, one ermine family defied its reputation and took up residence in my daughter, Bethany's, chicken coop for several years. They lived in harmony. There is no explanation for this other than Bethany's remarkable connection to animals. She told the ermines they could live there if they agreed not to bother the chickens.

Creatures of the Sky of Acadia National Park

Are you fascinated with the creatures of the sky? The birds, bees, butterflies, moths, bats, dragonflies, and a plethora of insects draw us out the door or to our windows to observe them. There are also those we hope to keep outside our screens. Regardless, we are entranced with their beauty, their variety, and their behavior. These airborne creatures offer opportunities for lifelong study and one more way to nurture something of the green outdoors. Latin names are included for some birds, other creatures, and plants in the next few sections. Challenging our minds to learn and remember these names is a great mental exercise.

BIRDS IN AND AROUND ACADIA NATIONAL PARK[56]
Thirty-six inches of snow in less than a week, after dramatic temperature swings and more than a month with no snow, seems shocking to the birds of Acadia. In sixty-knot gusts, we watch the crows and eagles blowing in the wind and the smaller birds unable to hang onto the branches and feeders. As the storm winds down, one exhausted junco collapses into the snow and remains there for too long. As I head out

the door to assist, it musters up its strength and flies into a leafy rhodo-dendron. The challenges faced by birds are great, particularly in winter. We do our best to augment their food supply; they provide an intimate view of nature from our kitchen window, making promises that they will be there for us during times when we cannot get out the door. Car-dinals, bluejays, chickadees, a downy woodpecker, juncos, and cedar waxwings provide colorful splashes against a cottony snow, seemingly appreciative of the berries and seeds that supply their fuel.

Birding is one of the fastest growing outdoor recreations. It is also one of the fastest growing segments of environmental research. Acadia National Park has long been an ideal location for bird research because it is a protected landscape on a major migratory corridor. The study of birds can teach lessons broadly applicable across the whole natural environment. For example, analyzing the changes in dates of arrival at Acadia National Park of a particular bird species may enable resource managers to anticipate future problems. If a bird species seems to be arriving increasingly early in the spring, that may suggest arrival before the maturing of a critical food that could lead to serious decline in population numbers with impacts throughout an ecosystem.

Decades before the term "citizen scientist" came into use, ama-teur birders at Acadia were recording their observations. Millions of migrating birds rely on downeast Maine's coastal and island habitats each spring and fall, and an impressive diversity of species breed or winter in the region's forests, on its islands, and in its waters. Climate change, land development, and wind energy facilities threaten many bird species. Acadia National Park possesses a wealth of invaluable related research and local historical records about birds that is heavily drawn upon by today's professional researchers and citizen scientists.

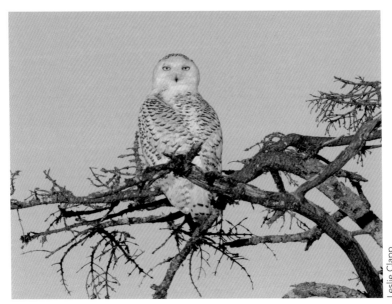

Leslie Clapp

Snowy Owl.

BIRDS OF ACADIA NATIONAL PARK (partial list)

There are 353 species of birds spotted in or around Acadia. This partial list includes birds I have seen, most of which are quite common. For some, my personal experience is added to inspire you to reflect on your own observations.

Bittern, American (*Botaurus lentiginosus*)
Phoebe Milliken, rightfully named, happens to be a bird-lover. One marvelous memory of a shared birding expedition at the Witch Hole Marsh found her excitedly hopping up and down whispering loudly, "Bittern, bittern! We must get closer." The steep bank and aging Phoebe were not a good combination. Her solution: sit down on the muddy bank in her pale blue pants and slide her way down to bittern land. Oh, what memories we have. Do you have a memory of a wildlife expedition with an older friend when you were both in a different place in life?

Crow, American (*Corvus brachyrhychos*)

We all know crows, but I have a story of a day with the crows that taught me a lesson.

The warm, pregnant fragrance of a humid spring day is filled with the scent of Miss Kim lilacs, decaying tulip petals, and the soft, sweet earth. My fingers dig deep into the dark soil to get the last of the stubborn mallow roots. Lovely in their designated home, they are quick to intrude upon their neighbors in their determination to propagate. Each spring their tap-rooted seedlings spring up everywhere despite our rigorous attempts to rid the parent plants of seed heads. This morning, I have yanked out dozens of little plants and dumped them onto the compost heap.

Phoebes sing their familiar message, and the wood thrush trills from its safe haven. A dozen fearless chickadees hop around me, searching for feeder spills as a ruby-throated hummingbird buzzes into the deep red of a Nova Zembla rhododendron. The baby crows and their eight adult family members chatter from the inner branches of the thick, old spruces that house their nests.

Crows aren't everyone's favorite bird, but I love this family and watch their antics through the seasons. They flap about and demand their rations each morning, shoving the smaller birds aside and fighting the squirrels for the tastier morsels. During the winter months, they depend upon our sacks of seed, perching in the bare maple branches or on our railing waiting for the meal delivery. Sometimes they are so piggy in their spring demands that they peck my hostas into strips and force me to move the winter feeders to the evergreen grove and away from my gardens. Once the whole group disappeared for a month, convincing me that a neighbor had done them in. Running along a stretch of undeveloped road one day, I heard what I was convinced were our crows and reassured myself that they had just moved. Then the whole group reappeared, hopping over our fields, sitting at attention in the tall trees around the gardens or flapping around the feeders, clearly assuming they were entitled to an endless supply of seed as they jabbered away at each other or at us.

On this spring morning, the steady crow chatter from the wooded hillside is transformed into desperate screeches of alarm. I wind my way out of the garden, careful not to step on small snapdragon seedlings or the acidanthera heads that poke up between the perennials, rounding the corner of the house just in time to see one of our resident bald eagles grabbing a baby crow from its nest as the adult crows attack from every direction. Their panicked shrieks and pecks do nothing to dissuade the eagle, who smoothly glides away. Five times he returns, plucking each baby crow from its nest, leaving the parents and the extended family to mourn their loss. Although I love the eagles and delight in their presence in this neighborhood, I am angry at them now—identifying with them as I flip to how I feel about cancer's attack on my child.

Later that day, I follow the sounds of robin trauma down the sloping field to the tree line at the ocean's edge. There I find the crows stealing away the baby robins as their frantic parents try to protect them. I turn, trudge back up the hill toward the house and reflect on my own mallow seedling destruction several hours earlier.

Gannet, Northern (*Morus bassanus*)
The gannet is an elegant large white seabird that can be spotted soaring gracefully over the waters of eastern Maine.

Goldfinch, American (*Spinus tristis*)
The bright yellow male goldfinch and his less colorful mate feed happily upon the thistles that grow in fields and along the shore.

Grosbeak, Rose-breasted (*Pheucticus ludovicianus*)
The lovely rose-breasted grosbeak, with its little parrot beak, was one of the first birds to catch my attention as a child.

Grouse, Ruffed (*Bonasa umbellus*)
Ruffed grouse can become as friendly as barnyard chickens. We have had up to three in residence in our snow-filled gardens for extended periods during the winter.

Guillemot, Black (*Cepphus grylle*)
The plump little guillemot seems a friendly bird as it visits alongside anchored boats.

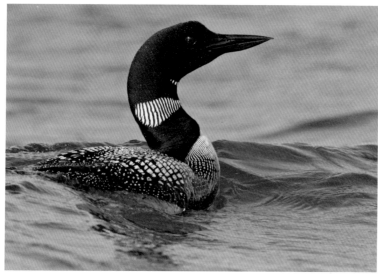

Leslie Clapp

Common Loon.

Gull, Herring (*Larus argentatus*)
Herring gulls abound on the Maine Coast, where they are frequently seen in large flocks.

Atlantic Puffin (*Fratercula arctica*)
Everyone loves a puffin, with its colorful bill and bold eyes. You can see them in the waters off Acadia National Park if you travel out into the ocean with Bar Harbor Whale Watch. Perhaps you remember Florence Page Jacques' poem, "Oh, there once was a puffin, just the shape of a muffin; And he lived on an island in the deep blue sea; He ate little fishes, that were most delicious; And he had them for breakfast and he had them for tea. ..."

In the Appendix to Chapter Seven, found on my website, you will find more members of the large troupe of Acadian birds that may pass through your area as well. Perhaps some of these are already your favorites. My pal, Sherry Streeter, is a great painter of birds and birds' nests with eggs. How do you express your love of the birds and other creatures?

POLLINATORS OF ACADIA NATIONAL PARK[82, 55, 57]
(partial list)

BATS AND OTHER VERTEBRATES

Bat, Eastern Small-Footed (*Myotis leibii*)

Bat, Little Brown (*Myotis lucifugus*)
Bats such as Acadia's Little Brown Bat and Large Brown Bat, are pollinators, as are other vertebrates including deer, rabbits, lizards, and rodents. Worldwide, more than 300 species of fruit and over 500 flowers depend upon bats as their exclusive or major pollinators.

BEES, WASPS, AND OTHER INSECTS (partial list)
More than 150 species of bees have been found in Acadia National Park.

Two-Spotted Bumblebee (*Bombus bimasculatus)*

Masked Bee (*Hyleaus basalis*) is uncommon in Acadia.

Metallic Sweat Bee (*Augochlorella aurata*) is a green bee.

Mining Bee (*Andrena frigida*), which is active in the spring, forages on spring-blooming plants.

Sweat Bee (*Lasioglossum leucocomum*) is a bee associated with sand.

Paper Wasps (*Vespula vulgaris*) have an unfair reputation, as they are one of the more docile wasps, unless bothered. My introduction to them came when I stepped on one at age four, an experience forever etched in my mind. Their beautiful hanging nests have individual egg cells, later filled with food for their young. Preferred foods are nectar and plant secretions, although they also prey on other insects.

BUTTERFLIES

Clouded Sulfur (*Colias philodice*) is a yellowish butterfly.

Eastern Tiger Swallowtail (*Papilioglaucus*) is a stunning large black and yellow creature.

Meadow Fritillary (*Boloria bellona*), often found in groups feeding in

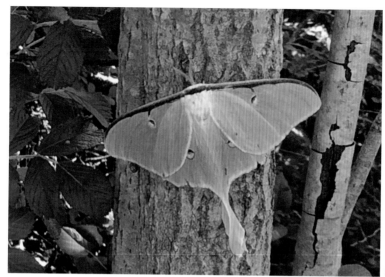

Dianna Emory

Luna Moth.

fields, resembles a small version of the monarch.

Monarch (*Danaus plexippus*) is a large black and orange striped butter-fly that is the most-celebrated of North American butterflies.

Mourning Cloak (*Nyphalis antiopa*) is a dark butterfly with iridescent blue spots along yellow-edged wings.

Red Admiral (*Vanessa atalanta*) is a black butterfly with four orange wing bands that has strong migration habits.

MOTHS

Achemon Sphinx Moth (*Eumorpha aschemon*) is a night moth with pink bands.

Banded Woollybear Caterpillar Moth (*Pyrrharctia isabella*) is loved for its bristly black and orange striped caterpillar.

Blinded Sphinx Moth (*Paonias excaecata*) is a fascinating shaggy moth that is easily camouflaged and is not blind.

Cecropia Silk Moth (*Hyalophora cecropia*) is North America's largest moth. It is soft as a feather.

Hummingbird Moth (*Hemaris sp.*) so much resembles a tiny hummingbird that it is often mistaken for a bird.

Luna Moth (*Actias luna*) is a large, elegant green moth that is always a treat to discover.

Promethea Moth (*Callosamia promethea*) is in the silkworm family.

Rosy Maple Moth (*Dryocampa rubicunda*) creates the silky cocoons found on maple trees.

(For additional lists, please see the Appendix to Chapter Seven on my website.)

HUMMINGBIRDS

Ruby-Throated Hummingbird (*Archilochus colubris*) is the beloved harbinger of late spring that returns each year to its summer home in the northeast. It is a wonderful pollinator.

Threats to Pollinators, Birds, Animals, and Plants

Developing an awareness of challenges to our natural world reminds us that we can assist in protection efforts. National park scientists and others are focused on key threats to pollinators. In addition to climate change and commercial production of monocrops, the destruction and fragmentation of natural habitat through excessive mowing of lawns and overweeding, particularly of blueberry farms, disrupts pollinators' access to food sources.

The systemic pesticides, neonicotinoids, are toxic to pollinators, including bees, flies, butterflies, moths, bats, and hummingbirds. These revolting chemicals are incorporated into plants and their flowers, where they are picked up by bees of all types in pollen and nectar. Despite compelling research, they are not banned by the EPA. Researchers from Pennsylvania State University have learned that plant odors modified by pollutants like ozone can confuse bees, "increasing the time bees must forage while decreasing their pollination efficiency and the amount of food they bring back to a colony."[46] Colony collapse disorder, which raises the mortality rate in honeybee hives, is linked to pesticides as well as diseases, pests, contemporary agricultural practices, and changes in the environment.

Researchers provide a wealth of information related to the devastating effects of climate change. Dr. Abe Miller-Rushing and his colleagues who work at Acadia National Park and Schoodic Institute observe the grave impact of environmental change and related ecological mismatches. Some of their shocking conclusions follow.

"Climate changes in the Acadia region have altered the populations and behaviors of species and have affected their interactions. Over the past 120 years, Acadia National Park has lost 18% of its native plant species" (Green et al. 2005).[47]

"Within the past 50 years, the Acadia region has gained more than 500 new insect species" (Chandler et al. 2012).[48]

"Within the past 50 years, the timing of bird migrations and breeding have changed throughout the Acadia region" (Miller-Rushing et al. 2008).[49]

"Climate changes may be creating mismatches among predators and prey, or plants and pollinators, by changing the timing of when various species depend on each others resources and services" (Miller-Rushing et al. 2008).[49]

"Ecological mismatches are one of the primary ways in which climate change is contributing to the decline and extinction of some plant and animal species" (Cahill et al. 2013).[50]

"Climate changes in precipitation and temperature cause shifts in flowering and fruiting of plant species. These shifts lead to flowers blooming before pollinators arrive. Birds find it difficult to find fruits to feed upon."[51]

In Chapter Ten, you will see what you can do to help to alleviate some of these problems.

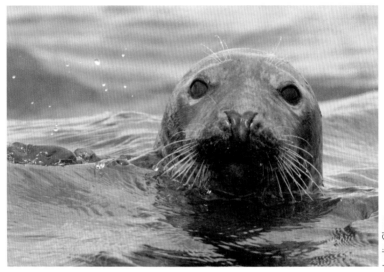

Leslie Clapp

Seal Looking at You.

Creatures of the Waters around Acadia National Park

The Appendix to Chapter Seven, found on my website, www.Dian-naEmory.com, provides a more extensive list of the marine mammals of the Acadia region. Fish and other marine creatures are so numerous that you are referred to other sources for complete lists. Some marine mammals that I have spotted from our boat or from the Bar Harbor Whale Watch vessel, with naturalist Zack Klyver's assistance, are:

MARINE MAMMALS (partial list)

Fin Whales (*Balaenoptera physalus*) are the second largest animal after the blue whale. They can be seen in the Acadia region on commercial whale watch trips, where naturalists are well-acquainted with these fast swimming "greyhounds of the sea."

Harbor Porpoises (*Phocoena phocoena*) are friendly creatures that are attracted to boat wakes, paddleboards, and other vessels. They seem curious about any sort of wake and regularly dive under my paddle-board and out of the water, crossing the bow of our boat.

Humpback Whales (*Megaptera novaeangliae*) are routinely seen from whale watch boats, where naturalists can identify individuals by their distinct markings. These large whales are quite acrobatic and provide impressive displays for viewers. One sail through Massachusetts Bay found us amidst hundreds of humpbacks, many of which spouted, breached, and rolled well into the night. Perhaps they were headed for the Acadia region.

Gray Seals (*Halichoerus grypus*), also known as horsehead seals, are land-breeding seals that are well-adapted for life in the North Atlantic. It is always a treat to interact with these large mammals, as they seem to observe us so closely.

Harbor Seals (*Phoca vitulina*) are a widely-distributed pinneped frequently seen in large packs hauled out on coastal ledges. It is not advisable to approach their ledges closely during pupping season, as it is disruptive to the herd. Seals are curious creatures that often follow small craft. I am still waiting for the day that one slides onto my paddleboard, which would be thrilling.

Also see Amphibians and Reptiles in the Creatures of the Lands section of Chapter Seven.

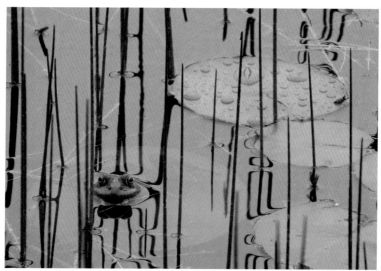

Melissa Savage

Frog and Lily Pads.

FLORA OF ACADIA NATIONAL PARK

"The Earth laughs in flowers."
Ralph Waldo Emerson

"Keep a green tree in your heart and perhaps a songbird will come."
Chinese Proverb

Like the creatures of our world, nature's flora can draw us in to a place where we want to learn more and more. Days exploring the forests and the fields, the bogs and the brooks, the shoreline and the waters, can introduce us to many species in their chosen environment. Evenings reading in a comfortable chair or at the computer give us access to details that can challenge our minds and keep us learning, regardless of what else is going on in our lives. The treasure trove of information that is available if one chooses to pursue it can help to blend enjoyment of wild flora, gardening, and indoor plant care, while encouraging us to consider all the ways we can satisfy our need for green space.

What you are provided here and in the Appendix to Chapter Seven, found on my website, represents some of the plants and trees that you can discover at Acadia and in much of the northeast. Eight hundred and sixty-two plants, or 41% of Maine's flora, were documented as occurring in Acadia National Park, according to *The Plants of Acadia National Park*,[52] a marvelous resource that Friends of Acadia, the Garden Club of Mount Desert, and the Maine Natural History Observatory helped produce with a team of talented botanists. Nineteen species are included in Maine's rare plant list. "Acadia National Park provides protected habitat vital to the persistence of these species within the region. In addition, Acadia National Park monitors the rare plant populations that occur on park lands and will conduct management activities if necessary to ensure their survival in the park."[52]

In the event that you decide to dig deeper into the world of plants in some way, perhaps you will choose to build a relationship with a particular patch of ground and its inhabitants, both flora and fauna, and watch it over time. Or, you may want to focus on an individual plant outdoors or indoors and begin to connect with it. The changes that you observe over time will amaze you. Although far from a botanist, I will pass on some nuggets of information gathered from many friends and other sources that I hope will inspire you to learn more. Latin names precede the common names in this section to challenge us to think first in Latin.

FLOWERING PLANTS AND SHRUBS
OF ACADIA NATIONAL PARK [58, 59] (partial list)

Amelanchier laevis (Smooth Shadbush): The most common shadbush in the three districts of Acadia, the alluring and delicate blossoms of the shad are harbingers of early spring.

Andromeda polifolia (Bog-rosemary): The little pink bells and stiff rosemary leaves of this bog plant always remind me of hikes at Schoodic, where you will readily find it.

Antennaria howellii (Small Pussytoes): Yes, they do look like my white kitty's toes as they scatter themselves around rocky, thin-soiled areas.

Arisaema triphyllum (Jack-in-the-Pulpit): Although uncommon in Acadia, I cannot resist listing this perky plant with its surprising striped blossom.

Asclepias syriaca (Common Milkweed): Oh, how we love the fragrant stands of these pink blossoms that evolve into hair-filled pods. Uncommon in Acadia, they are the favorite food of the endangered monarch butterfly. We plant the annual species in our gardens to encourage the monarchs.

Calystegia sepium (Hedge Bindweed): Wild pink morning glories wind their vines along the edges of ocean beaches.

Chamaepericlymenum canadense (Bunchberry): The four-petaled white blossoms and red berry clusters of this herb are scattered in large swaths over blueberry barrens and woodlands.

Daucus carota (Queen Anne's Lace): Flat, airy white blossoms wave in the breezes from wildflower fields.

Epigaea repens (Trailing Arbutus): Fragrant pink mayflowers with their glossy, oval leaves are found growing thickly on dry banks, wooded areas, and our leachfield.

Eurybia macrophylla (Large-leafed Aster): Pale purple florets of this herb abound in forested areas of the Park.

Gaylussacia baccata (Black Huckleberry): An edible, but very seedy, berry adorns this bushy shrub.

Gaultheria procumbens (Wintergreen): The wintergreen-flavored red berries and leaves of this short woodland shrub are often found in mossy areas.

Fragaria virginiana (Wild Strawberry): June fields reveal first delicate white blossoms, then tiny, luscious strawberries.

Hieracium aurantiacum (Devil's Paint-brush): Eye-catching orange-red flowers adorn the hairy stems of these common field flowers.

Houstonia caerulea (Bluets): Tiny blue four-petaled blossoms with yellow eyes pop up in fields and on lawns as a promise of early summer.

Ilex verticillata (Winterberry): Winter's wet areas come alive with the alluring red berries of this alder bush.

Iris hookeri (Arctic Blue Flag): A large stand of this treasured species is found on Schoodic's Moose Island.

Iris versicolor (Larger Blue Flag): This common iris is abundant in fresh water wetlands, producing a spectacular springtime display.

Kalmia angustifolia (Sheep Laurel): Bright pink bells catch one's attention on hillsides and in wet areas.

Lathyrus japonicas (Beach-pea): With its lovely blue flowers and pea-pods, it winds itself along the sandy and rocky edges of ocean beaches.

Leucanthemum vulgare (Ox-eye Daisy): Scores of these familiar white daisies fill the fields and disturbed areas of Acadia, delighting all.

Limonium carolinianum (Sea-lavender): The shores of Mount Desert and the Schoodic District are home to this noticeable branched lavender herb.

Linaria vulgaris (Butter and Eggs): True to the colors of its name, common toadflax finds its home on roadsides and disturbed areas.

Lysimachia borealis (Starflower): Seven-petaled stars rest within a nest of pointed leaves on this forest herb.

Monitropa uniflora (Indian Pipe): Magical when found springing forth in the rich woods, the poisonous pipes are also known as convulsion-root and corpse-plant.

Ranunculus acris (Tall Buttercup): Disturbed areas attract these branching yellow-flowered plants, which are poisonous to some livestock.

Rhus typhina (Staghorn Sumac): Gorgeous, velvety burgundy spires distinguish this common shrub that is often seen in large stands on roadsides and in open areas.

Rhododendron canadense (Rhodora): The beloved purple blossoms of the rhodora emerge before its leaves and are a harbinger of Acadia's spring.

Rosa rugosa (Salt-spray Rose): Lovely on coastal beaches or cultivated hedgerows, when planted in gardens Rosa rugosa is a nightmare to remove.

Rosa virginiana (Virginia Rose): Common to all districts of Acadia, this pale pink rose frequents dry marshes.

Rudbeckia hirta (Black-eyed Susan): Hairy stems support yellowish-orange heads of these coneflowers.

Salix discolor (Pussy Willow): Born in wet areas, this tall shrub sports soft gray pussies that burst into greenish-yellow fuzzies.

Sambucus racemosa (Red Elderberry): Fire engine red inedible berries appear in early summer following lovely white clusters on these tall shrubs.

Solidago Canadensis (Canada Goldenrod): The most common of the many goldenrods found in Acadia, its easily-recognizable late summer heads mark a turn toward fall.

Symplocarpus foetidus (Eastern Skunk-cabbage): Found easily on Isle au Haut, this purple-blossomed swamp plant with its stinky odor and

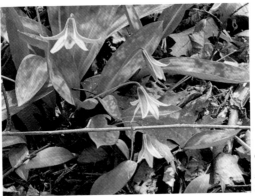

Trout Lilies.

large leaves is uncommon on MDI.

Symphyotrichum novi-belgii (New York Aster): Yellow-eyed purple blossoms adorn this common coastal flower.

Tanacetum vulgare (Common Tansy): A fragrant herb, this yellow-headed perennial is lovely enough for even the fanciest gardens.

Taraxacum officinale (Common Dandelion): The bane of the perfect lawn-minded, the familiar fluffy yellow blossoms of this plant are a favorite food of honey bees and should be left unmowed when possible.

Typha latifolia (Broad-leaved Cat-tail): Sporting tall, thin, upright brown "tails," this herb forms large stands in marshes.

Vaccinium augustifolium (Lowbush Blueberry): Scattered over the mountains and valleys of Acadia National Park, blueberries are a cook's favorite for pies and muffins.

Vaccinium vitis-idaea (Mountain Cranberry): Thick patches of these lingonberries cover the edges of granite shores on many of Acadia's easement islands.

Vicia cracca (Cow Vetch): This purple-blossomed vetch is so lovely that it is allowed to wind its way throughout my gardens when it chooses.

Viola cucullata (Marsh Blue Violet): Found in wet areas, this pale purple violet distinguishes itself through its location.

Viola pallens (Northern White Violet): The most common of the white violets in Acadia, this species is found in wet areas.

Viola sororia (Wooly Blue Violet): All districts of Acadia hold this woodland and meadow violet.

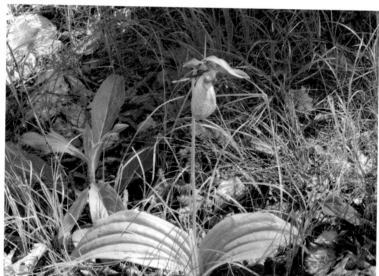

Pink Lady's Slipper.

Melissa Savage

ORCHIDS

Orchids are listed separately for your pleasure in the pursuit of these beloved blooms.

Arethusa bulbosa (Dragon's Mouth): This swamp pink has one exquisite flower per stem.

Calopogon tuberosus (Grass Pink): An orchid found in wet meadows, this herb sports hot pink flowers with fuzzy yellow tops.

Cypripedium acaule (Pink Lady's Slipper): The largest stand of this amazing plant that I have seen in or around Acadia is at the wooded entrance to our friends' home, which is frequently shared on the Garden Club of Mount Desert's Garden Tour.

Pogonia ophioglossoides (Rose Pogonia): The bogs of Isle au Haut are a frequent home to these yellow-lipped pink orchids.

Platanthera lacera (Ragged Fringed Orchid): Rare to Acadia, we treasure an extensive stand of these lovely orchids that are scattered about in our Sedgwick farm's meadows.

FERNS, SEDGES, GRASSES, AND RUSHES

The numerous ferns, sedges, grasses, and rushes of Acadia will be left for your own exploration.

TREES OF ACADIA NATIONAL PARK[60] (partial list)

Abies balsamea (Balsam Fir): The most abundant evergreen conifer in Maine, this fragrant traditional Christmas tree is often found in the damp woods of Acadia.

Acer rubrum (Red Maple): The swamp maple, which typically does not have a divided trunk, is the most abundant of the maples.

Acer saccharum (Sugar Maple): Autumn brings shades of red, orange, yellow, and scarlet to the leaves of the sugar maple, while late winter brings the promise of maple syrup days.

Betula alleghaniensis (Yellow Birch): Distinguished by its yellow peeling bark, this is the largest of the birches, growing up to 30 meters.

Betula papyrifera (White Birch): Also known to me as paper birch and canoe birch, this is the tree renowned for the building of birch bark canoes by Native Americans.

Betula populifolia (Gray Birch): This short-lived birch of up to 10 meters has a shinier leaf with a longer point than other birches and does not exfoliate its bark.

Fagus grandifolia (American Beech): Beech, which produce edible nuts in a burr, can be found in nearly pure stands with dead leaves remaining through winter.

Picea glauca (White Spruce): Also called the cat spruce, the evergreen needles have the fragrance of cat urine, thus these trees are not recommended as Christmas trees. White spruce will not tolerate shade and is often found in open areas.

Picea rubens (Red Spruce): This evergreen is commonly found growing in well-drained rocky soils in the forests of all districts of Acadia, particularly on the north mountain slopes.

Pinus banksiana (Jack Pine): Acadia's Schoodic District hosts the most significant stand of this short-needled pine which grows in sandy, rocky soil.

Pinus resinosa (Red Pine): Also known as Norway pine, red pine sports two-needled clusters and is typically found in sandy or dry soil.

Pinus rigida (Pitch Pine): Growing in gravelly sandy soil, this pine is distinguished by its clusters of three needles and the fact that "it is the only native pine that is distinguished by sprout growth."[60]

Pinus strobus (White Pine): Soft five-needled clusters distinguish this lovely pine that is common to all Park districts.

Populus tremuloides (Quaking Aspen): Underground shoots are usually responsible for the reproduction of this smooth, gray-barked aspen that is often the first species to establish after fires or clear cuts.

Thuja occidentalis (Northern White Cedar): Also known as Eastern arborvitae, this fragrant cedar is found in moist areas. Its broad, flat evergreen leaves are a special treat for white-tailed deer.

Tsuga Canadensis (Eastern Hemlock): Not found in the Schoodic District, this evergreen is distinguished by its scaly bark and short, flat, blunt needles.

Quercus rubra (Northern Red Oak): Found in the Mount Desert and Isle au Haut Districts of Acadia, this tall oak bears acorns, a prized food of squirrels and other small mammals.

PLANTS OF THE WATERS IN AND AROUND
ACADIA NATIONAL PARK (partial list)

As you hike along the shorelines of the Maine coast, one of the most noticeable plants you will find is rockweed (*Ascophyllum nodosum*), a marine alga. When the tide is in, rockweed waves from where it grows from rocks on the ocean floor, while low tide finds it laid in clumps along the shore. Several years ago, we were horrified to watch harvesters ripping the rockweed from the shoreline of The Nature Conservancy's Great Wass Island in eastern Maine. Rockweed is prized as a fertilizer, and some short-sighted harvesters have ignored guidelines for trimming the weed, which cannot recover if it is ripped off the rocks. Rockweed is protected in the national park, as are all other plants found there, and is also of concern to many landowners.

The salt waters find other types of seaweeds and kelps floating or rooted to the ocean floor, serving as safe havens for small fish, crustaceans, and other creatures.

Among the eighty plus freshwater (aquatic) plants in Acadia National Park are the water lilies found in shades of pink, white, and yellow. As one examines them, it is not unusual to find a turtle's nose poking through the water's surface, frogs perched upon the lily pads, or other creatures hiding amidst their roots.

THE THREAT OF INVASIVE PLANTS

As climate change increasingly allows the winter survival of annual exotics, numerous invasive plants are threatening the native vegetation of Acadia, as well as of your own region. Unwittingly, businesses and individuals have transported invasive plants for landscaping and garden specimens. Many of the shrubby species produce fruits that are consumed by birds, with the seeds then scattered about to choke out native species. One example is Japanese barberry, which also is prime habitat for the deer ticks that transmit Lyme disease, according to Jeffrey Ward, chief scientist in the forestry and horticultural department at the Connecticut Agricultural Experiment Station.

Boaters and fishermen have also brought invasive plants to the area on their boats' bottoms. These invasive plants can be "so fast-growing and aggressive that they crowd out and even eliminate natives, resulting in plant communities that comprise only a few species."[52]

The National Wildlife Federation mentions that Japanese knotweed has "crowded out indigenous vegetation eaten by invertebrates, and scientists suspect that the loss of these animals may, in turn, be starving green frogs."[53] Another culprit is the Asian imported kousa dogwood, thought to have introduced the fungal disease that has decimated native flowering dogwoods that produce berries rich in calcium beneficial to birds and mammals. The fruit of kousa dogwood, in contrast, produces nothing edible for North American wildlife, according to Doug Tallamy, a University of Delaware professor of wildlife ecology and entomology whom my garden club was fortunate to have as a speaker.[54]

As you can well imagine, there is plenty of room for a host of volunteers to eradicate invasives and to educate others about species such as the kousa dogwood, topics we will pursue in Chapter Ten.

INVASIVE PLANTS OF ACADIA NATIONAL PARK[55]
(partial list)

Acer platanoides (Norway Maple)

Alliaria petoilata (Garlic Mustard)

Berberis thunbergii (Japanese Barberry)

Celastrus orbiculatus (Oriental Bittersweet)

Euonymus alatus (Winged Euonymus)

Frangula alnus (Glossy Buckthorn)

Lonicera (Nonnative Honeysuckle)

Lythrum salicaria (Purple Loosestrife)

Rosa multiflora (Multiflora Rose)

Reynoutria japonica (Japanese Knotweed)

Solanum dulcamara (Deadly Nightshade) note: all parts of this plant are poisonous.

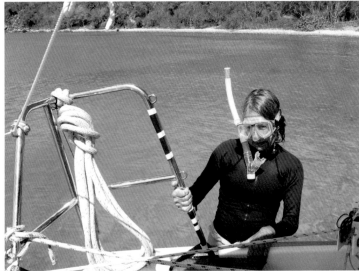

Ben Emory

Emerging from Magical Waters.

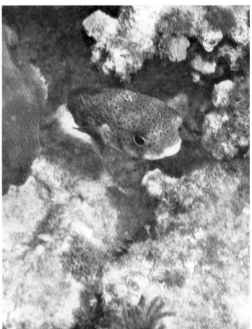

Dianna Emory

An Engaging Porcupinefish.

8

VENTURING FORTH INTO
VIRGIN ISLANDS NATIONAL PARK

"Nature will bear the closest inspection.
She invites us to lay our eye level with her smallest leaf
and take an insect view of its plain."
Henry David Thoreau

Sometimes the place to which we count on venturing forth needs to heal, as is the case with the Virgin Islands National Park in the wake of Hurricane Irma. I have written of that in the Post-Hurricane Tribute to Virgin Islands National Park. Found below is a description of an intact St. John. We count upon our memories and our imaginations to take us there during the period of healing that lies ahead. Chapter Eight is also offered as a reminder of what we are at risk of losing in this world.

The opportunity to retreat to our federal lands holds anticipation and relief. Summer's heat inspires us to head for the shorelines of the nation's fresh and salt waters or crisp days in the mountains. Dark days and the depths of winter conjure up dreams of sugar sand, warm breezes, tropic waters, and a host of undersea adventures. How we long for those nurturing temperatures—the cool ones we seek in the summer and the warmth offering respite from winter's icy grasp. Virgin Islands National Park (VINP) offers the perfect destination for those seeking a tropic adventure replete with plenty of hiking, snorkeling, swimming, sailing, and other water-based activities. We will focus on the St. John component of VINP as an example of building a repertoire of experiences and visual images of the tropics and its creatures.

BACKGROUND INFORMATION

More than two-thirds of the twenty square mile island of St. John, which is part of a vast underwater mountain range, is protected by Virgin

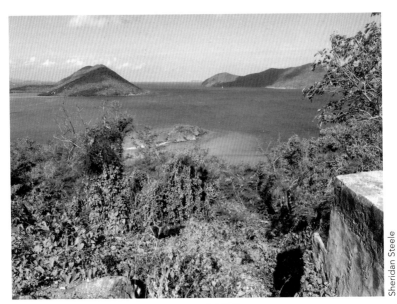

America Hill, VINP.

Sheridan Steele

Islands National Park. Much of the land in the Park was donated by Laurance Rockefeller when it was established in 1956. Since that time more land has been added, including the 2008 addition of the Maho Bay watershed with the assistance of the Trust for Public Land and the 2017 donation of additional nearby acreage by a private philanthropist.

Sub-tropical in climate and located in the path of the balmy trade winds, St. John provides great variation in rainfall. Forests cover 85.5% of the island. Its southeast side, near the Ram's Head section of the Park, is arid and dry, supporting cacti and other dry-climate plants. The north side of the island from Caneel Bay to East End and Haulover Bay is heavily forested, mountainous, and supports wet-tropical vegetation. Soils are volcanic in origin, thus acidic. Most of St. John's vegetation is secondary forest that continues to recover from the deforestation of 90% of the vegetation for Danish plantation agriculture in the 1800's.

Virgin Islands National Park is assisted in its efforts by Friends of VINP, Virgin Islands Environmental Research Station (VIERS), Trust for Public Lands (TPL), The Nature Conservancy (TNC), and other partners.

THE LANDS OF VIRGIN ISLANDS
NATIONAL PARK

Hiking and Running VINP

The mountainous and rocky nature of VINP and the traffic activity on the roads of St. John discourage biking, but the island is a runner's and hiker's ideal destination. The hot temperatures require careful hydration, and the lack of access to supplies or medical assistance from many locations in the Park is underscored. Those respectful of the climate, terrain, and, of course, the environment, are in for a treat.

Over the years, we have greatly enjoyed hiking VINP's trail network, leading to a strong list of favorites. For detailed assistance, Gerald Singer has produced the outstanding guidebook, *St. John Off the Beaten Track*,[61] and Bob Garrison markets the excellent *The Last Trail Bandit Guide to the Hiking Trails of St. John, VI*,[62] which shares information beyond what is found in the very good VINP materials.

Many days one can combine a long hike with a swim and a snorkel or two. Beginning at Francis Bay, follow the nature trail for good birding along the shores of the salt ponds. This in itself is a good beginner trail that also provides handicapped access. A walk along the road and through mangrove arches takes one to the shore trail to Leinster Bay's Waterlemon Cay, one of the best snorkeling expeditions around for the timid or the tough. There you will often see turtles, a family of spotted eagle rays, and a multitude of fish. Snorkeling around Waterlemon Cay ensures encounters with many more fish, rays, corals, sponges, and large starfish. A strong current can exist in the cut, so inexperienced swimmers should wear fins. Following your expedition there, head again for the hiking and follow the Johnny Horn Trail to the turn to Brown Bay. On the Brown Bay trail, a magnificent salt pond provides great views of stilts and great egrets, whose rookery is nearby. Off come the hiking shoes again at Brown Bay for the best of the VINP snorkeling, in our opinion. The western side of Brown Bay bears exploring on foot, as it is covered with ruins that take one back to an earlier time in St. John's history.

The Brown Bay expedition can be shortened if a car awaits you

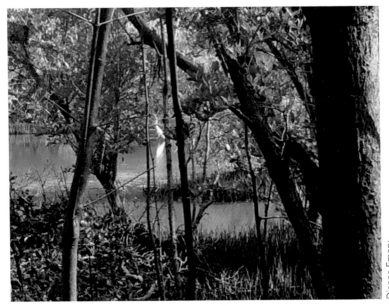

Dianna Emory

Great Egret Rookery.

back on the main road, accessed via the remainder of the trail. We prefer, however, to stay on our feet and do the loop that takes you along the road past Estate Zootenvale and into Coral Bay. The return to the Johnny Horn Trail and Leinster Bay begins at the Moravian Church—or perhaps you will take a side trip into Coral Bay for lunch or provisions to stuff into your backpacks.

As I have described this hike/run/snorkel combo, memories have taken me right back there. My mind's eye is filled with individual fish that inhabit different parts of the reefs, land crabs rolling down hillsides, merry chirps of stilts as they feed in the salt pond, the scent of decaying forest vegetation, and the transition from a sweaty mess to an unencumbered swimmer who streaks through refreshing waters amidst the ocean's creatures. How easy it is to recall our favorite places and experiences, immerse in their detail, and carry ourselves to a comfortable space in our memories or imaginations.

How about taking yourself to one of those places for a few moments right now? Just close your eyes and let yourself drift to that special place for a few moments. Rest and relax there, enjoying the sights, the sounds, the scents, and all else that you feel or sense. Breathe deeply of inner peace, comfort, and relaxation and then open your eyes.

THE WATERS AROUND VIRGIN ISLANDS NATIONAL PARK

Swimming
The Virgin Islands provide the most relaxing and safe swimming of anywhere in the Eastern Caribbean, with gentle beaches where children and the elderly can ease themselves into the water, as well as challenging long-distance swims around exposed reefs. Each year, Friends of the Virgin Islands National Park and others produce a benefit swimming marathon that draws the courageous. They swim from Maho Beach to Hawksnest Beach, a distance of 3.5 miles. Other courses and team swims are also offered. Join a team and build some friendships in a new way.

Snorkeling and Diving
Early in this book, you read several visualizations that relate to snorkeling adventures. I hope that you will find yourself snorkeling or diving in the Virgin Islands one day or enjoying videos of the scenery and living things that are there. Even if you are confined to a bed and very old, I think you will find that watching footage of experiences in the Virgin Islands National Park will captivate you and help you to create visualizations of miraculous creatures under the sea. Perhaps you would like to choose one and study it in great detail. I would choose the octopus or maybe the squid. Well, maybe the spotted trunk fish, or the green turtle, or the stoplight parrotfish, or the fairy baslet…

You could snorkel or dive every day of your life and still find something thrilling. It is the best way to bond with the ocean and her creatures, while exploring the waters that make up most of our world. What you will find there will transport you through time and space to a marvelous sea that is home to thousands of fish, corals, sponges, grasses, mammals, and other living things. Some people may be anxious about the risk of encountering dangerous creatures, but the worry of aggressive sharks or barracudas is over-dramatized. If you see a shark other than a docile nurse shark, which would be surprising, just return slowly to shore or your boat. Barracudas are not dangerous. They are curious. Remove your jewelry so that it does not look like a fishing lure. Do not stand on or touch corals, which can cut you and hurt the corals. No grabbing moray eels, urchins, or jellyfish, and no sticking your hands into holes. Actually, it is important that you keep your hands off marine life in general. These are living creatures, and you are in their home. Please care for them. To protect yourself from the greatest danger, avoid swimming in boat traffic. Wear a flag that helps others to see you, or wind some fluorescent tape around the top of your snorkel. Be aware of currents, and observe Park notices of swimming conditions. There are many guidebooks that suggest snorkeling spots. Our favorites include Little Lameshur Bay, Great Lameshur Bay, East End, Leinster Bay, Caneel Bay, Hawksnest Bay, and Brown Bay.

Sailing, Powerboating, Stand-up Paddle Boarding, Rowing, and Kayaking

Because I am a water enthusiast, I could speak for hours about the merits of various types of watercraft and how getting out on the water gives you a different perspective on the land that you have explored. It is amazing to skim along the water's surface in any craft, absorbing all that is around you. Perusing the land base and seeing geological features from the water give you an entirely difference perspective as you look at the mountain you climbed; the woods you explored; the ledges and reefs that hold caves you would like to know; and the sensitive or heedless placement of structures in the midst of nature. It also makes you think about the history of the place and how you can make a difference during your little pocket of time in the world.

Kayaks are abundant in the tropics, providing opportunities for exploration of places not accessible by bigger boats. They are rented in various locations around St. John, including at the National Park's Honeymoon Beach and Cinnamon Bay, where plastic and fiberglass

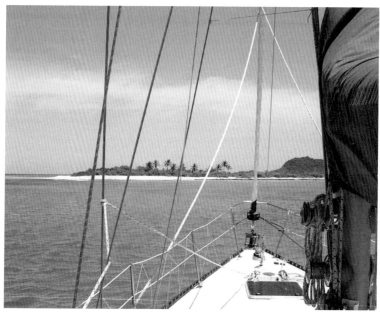

The Oceans Bind Us All Together.

Ben Emory

paddleboards are also available. Plastic paddle boards and kayaks are quite stable, but the beginner should plan to head upwind first. The downwind ride can seem easy, and you don't want to be shocked when you need to turn around and head in the opposite direction. Winds can come up quickly in the Virgins, and tacking across the wind, instead of paddling straight into it, is much easier. If you have trouble on a paddle board, get down onto your knees and keep moving. Getting wet in tropic waters is not so bad, and you will have a wonderful experience exploring the nooks and crannies that others can't reach. Private companies can instruct you or arrange tours.

Powerboats, windsurfers, dinghies, and small sailboats can be rented on St. John. Day and overnight charters can be arranged on St. John and cruising boats can be chartered for longer adventures, including to the U.S. Virgin Islands National Park, through numerous companies on nearby Tortola, British Virgin Islands.

FAUNA OF VIRGIN ISLANDS NATIONAL PARK

The lands, the sky, and the waters of the tropics are home to so many creatures. Many live beneath the surface of the sea. Endless opportunities exist to bond with a host of creatures, whether through direct contact or research. You are encouraged to get to know some of them well, to incorporate them into your thinking and visualizations, and to bring them into your life in whatever way you can. To challenge our minds, Latin names are included for many species.

As I contemplate the aging process or reflect upon the times that I have been infirmed, the importance of visions of underwater flora and fauna come to my mind. Have you noticed the calming influence of tropical fish drifting around their tank in your dentist's office or a video of undersea life that offers distraction during the wait for the doctor's appointment? Whether you have experienced them first-hand in the ocean or in aquariums or videos, there is something about the waving flora and drifting fish of the tropics that is mesmerizing. The visualizations I employ when I am in the most difficult of circumstances use imagery of these creatures. References to tropic flora and fauna have proved effective with scores of patients, regardless of whether they have ever made a trip to that world. Right now, can you close your eyes and conjure up an image of a tropical fish? Can you see the details of the plants around that fish as they wave in the currents of the water?

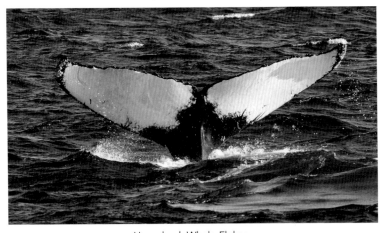

Humpback Whale Flukes.

Leslie Clapp

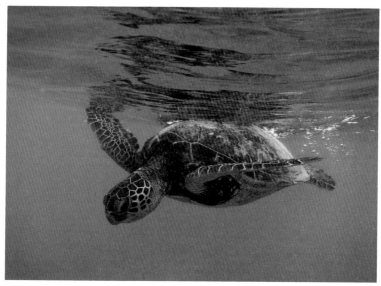

Leslie Clapp

Green Sea Turtle.

Creatures of the Lands of Virgin Islands National Park[72]

REPTILES (partial list)

Green Iguana (*Iguana iguana*)

Green Iguanas range in color from bright green babies to brown, black, or dark green adults that can grow to four feet in length. They are found basking in the sun or grazing on tasty vegetation, particularly on the lawns of the St. John Westin, where dozens are protected. At dusk, they climb high into the palms or canopy. Iguanas are fascinating animals that have keen eyesight, move quickly, and can bite. I can verify the biting. We housed daughter Bethany's iguanas, Lettuce and Tomato, while she lived in Spain after college. Feeding and cage cleaning were a challenge. Despite that, I love iguanas and particularly enjoy the memory of dozens of them charging down a Bahamian beach to meet our dinghy. When we climbed out and approached them, the entire herd took off at high speed in the opposite direction, only to turn and charge toward us once more when we stopped.

AMPHIBIANS (partial list)

Antillean Frog (*Eleutherodactylus antillensis*) is a forest frog that has dark spotted thighs, cinnamon eyes, and sings "churee-churee."

Cuban Tree Frog (*Osteopilus septentrionalis*) is a partially web-footed, 3-5 inch frog whose skin mucous causes temporary redness, itching, and swelling in humans. Considered invasive, they eat the local tree frogs.

Local Tree Frog, for which I find no Latin name, is a tiny frog, not much bigger than a dime, that sings in the same sequence with large numbers of its friends when it is wet outside.

Puerto Rican Whistling Eleuth (*Eleutherodactylus cochranae)* emits a long, piercing whistle followed by clicks.

CRUSTACEANS (partial list)

Caribbean Hermit Crab (*Coenobita clypeatus*) is a land crab that lives in the shells of other creatures and mass-migrates to the sea each year to deposit its eggs. When hiking, you will frequently find them rolling down the trail.

Land Crab (*Cardisoma guanhumi*) is a burrow-dwelling crab reaching 4-5 inches, excluding its claws. Its huge holes are found in many places in VINP. Occasionally, you will be lucky enough to see a crab.

SNAKES, all non-poisonous (partial list)

Blind Snake (*Typhlops richardii*)

Garden Snake (*Magliophis exiggum*) is the only snake I have ever spotted on St. John. Each time, it has been near the Lind Point Trail in the Park.

MAMMALS (partial list)

Representatives of the twenty-two species of mammals found in Virgin Islands National Park are interesting characters. The only mammal native to St. John is the bat, according to VINP. Deer are seen occasionally. The donkeys, sheep, and goats of St. John are notorious for their forays along beaches, roads, and hiking trails. Cats and dogs are also abundant. The local animal shelter appreciates your help with their

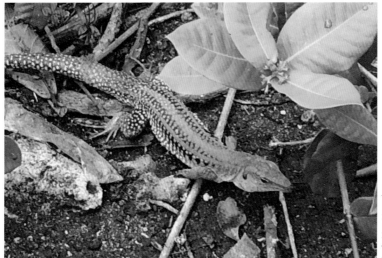

Flora and Fauna.

Cody Van Heerden

needs. The Reef Bay Trail is a place where we have spotted large boars and regularly seen evidence of pigs rooting in the earth. Unfortunately, mongoose have considerably impacted the bird population. They are cute like a ferret, but an unwelcome resident of the Park. We have spotted no rats.

Black Rat***
Deer
Donkey
Goat
Mongoose***
Norway Rat***
Pig
Sheep
***Exotic Invasive Species "are responsible for the extinction of multiple species of mammals, birds, reptiles, invertebrates, and plants and are particularly damaging to the flora and fauna of islands," according to the Virgin Islands Department of Agriculture, Forestry Division.

Creatures of the Sky of Virgin Islands National Park

BIRDS OF VIRGIN ISLANDS
NATIONAL PARK AND ST. JOHN[84]

St. John is home to over 140 species of birds including two species of hummingbirds, neither of which is found in the continental United States. The greatest threat is to ground birds, like doves, that are prey of the mongoose. Additional birds are listed in the Appendix to Chapter Eight on my website. Below you will find some of my favorites.

American Oystercatcher (*Haematopus palliates*) is found wintering along marshes and shores in the Virgin Islands, where it eats bivalves.

Bananaquit (*Coereba flaveola*) is a nectar-loving bird that is widespread on St. John.

Belted Kingfisher (*Megaceryle alcyon*) is found nesting in earthy burrows along the shore. Their noticeable call is frequent as they hover over water and plunge for fish.

Black-Necked Stilt (*Himantopus mexicanus*) is a common shorebird with red legs and striking black and white plumage.

Bobolink (*Dolichonyx oryzivorus*), easily distinguished by its bold black and white suit and yellow cap, migrates from the northern and northeastern United States through the Virgin Islands and on to South America.

Brown Booby (*Sula leucogaster*) is an entertaining seabird seen often around St. John. When fishing, it plummets straight into the water.

Brown Pelican (*Pelecanus occidentalis*) is found year-round in the Virgin Islands. As Dixon Lanier Merritt noted, "What a wonderful bird is the pelican. His bill can hold more than his belly can. He can hold in his beak enough food for a week! But I'll be darned if I know how the hellican?"

Great Blue Heron (*Ardea herodias*), the largest of the herons, winters in the Virgin Islands and is easily spotted by its size, stately motionless stance, and tucked neck when flying.

Great Egret (*Ardea alba*) is a large and stunning year-round white wading bird.

Magnificent Frigatebird (*Fregata magnificens*) is often seen silhouetted high in the sky, looking kite-like.

Pearly-Eyed Thrasher (*Margarops fuscatus*) often finds itself on your table eyeing your sandwich.

Red-Billed Tropicbird (*Phaethon aethereus*) is a lovely long-tailed seabird with a distinct red bill.

Royal Tern (*Thalasseus maximus*) is a striking orange-beaked and crested bird with a memorable call that is found year-round along Virgin Island beaches.

Smooth-Billed Ani (*Crotophaga ani*) is a gregarious bird in the cuckoo family with an entertaining call that greets hikers when they approach.

POLLINATORS OF VIRGIN ISLANDS NATIONAL PARK AND ST. JOHN[72] (partial list)

BATS AND OTHER VERTEBRATES

If you examine the ceilings of ruins on St. John, you could have the treat of finding bats in their home.

Mexican Fruit Bat (*Artibeus jamaicensis*)

Antillean Fruit-Eating Bat (*Brachyphylla cavernarum*)

Fishing Bat (*Noctilio leporinus*)

Velvety Free-Tailed Bat (*Molossus molossus*)

Red Fruit Bat (*Stenoderma rufum*)

Mexican Free-Tailed Bat (*Tadarida brasiliensis*)

BEES, WASPS, FLIES, AND OTHER INSECTS

There are many species of invaluable pollinators, including bees, wasps, flies, and other insects. The troublesome mosquitoes, biting flies, and the no-see-ums feed the bats and the birds, which justifies their usefulness.

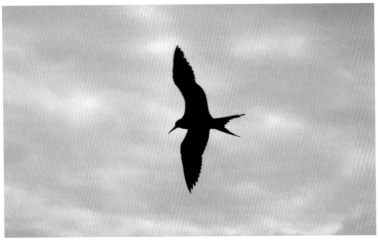

Dianna Emory

Frigate Bird in Flight.

Take bug spray when hiking or beaching to protect you from bites.

BUTTERFLIES AND MOTHS

Gulf Fritillary (*Agraulis vanillae*), also known as the passion butterfly, is a reddish-orange butterfly with black spots.

Monarch (*Danaus plexippus*) is a large, endangered milkweed-feeding butterfly that is orange with black stripes and outlines.

Great Southern White (*Ascia monuste*) is a small, white butterfly that is often seen in groups. Females are off-white to gray.

Cloudless Sulfur (*Phoebis sennae*) is a medium-sized, yellowish common butterfly.

Zebra (*Heliconius charithonia*) is a common black butterfly with white or yellowish stripes.

HUMMINGBIRDS

Antillean Crested Hummingbird (*Orthorhyncus cristatus*) sports a green crest that extends to its beak.

Green-throated Carib (*Eulampis holosericeus*) has a distinctly green head, banded with blue.

Creatures of the Waters of Virgin Islands National Park[63, 64, 65, 66]

Visions of the Virgin Islands often include some of the 302 species of fish found in their turquoise seas. More than fifty corals and a great variety of sponges and gorgonians also inhabit the waters. Below are some common and engaging reef fish and other creatures. Open ocean and fresh water creatures are left to your own research. More reef fish and reef creature species are found in the Appendix to Chapter Eight, found on my website, www.DiannaEmory.com.

REEF FISH (partial list of my favorites)

Blue Chromis (*Chromis cyanea*) is a common, bright blue fish with a deeply forked tail. 3-4 inches.

Blue Tang (*Acanthurus coeruleus*) is a pale to dark blue fish most often seen in large schools that drift en masse. 5-10 inches.

Fairy Basslet (*Gramma loretto*) is a striking bi-colored fish with a purple front and yellow rear. We have followed colonies of these little fish for years. 2-3 inches.

Gray Angelfish (*Pomacanthus arcuatus*) is a gray disk-shaped angel with yellow accents. 8-14 inches.

Queen Angelfish (*Holacanthus ciliaris*) is a large disk-shaped nearly iridescent greenish-blue angel with yellow fins. 10-18 inches.

Redlip Blenny (*Ophioblennius macclurei*) rests on rocks or reefs with its bulging eyes and red smiling lips. 2.5-4.5 inches.

Rock Beauty (*Holacanthus tricolor*) is a disk-shaped fish with a bright yellow front and tail, black sides, and blue lips. 5-8 inches.

Sergeant Major (*Abudefduf saxatilis*) is a gregarious silver fish with black stripes and yellow accents. 4-6 inches.

Scrawled Filefish (*Aluterus scriptus*) is a tan-to-gold fish with bluish green spots and markings. The lips protrude and the tail is broom-like. 12-30 inches.

Smooth Trunkfish (*Lactophyrus triqueter*) is a blackish odd-shaped fish covered with spots. Its eyes protrude, as does its mouth. 6-10 inches.

Spotted Drum (*Equetus punctatus*) is not common but is a favorite fish that I see regularly on one reef. He is quite remarkable, and I hope you see him around his cave. 6-9 inches.

Squirrelfish (*Holocentrus adscensionis*) is a big-eyed reddish fish with a spiny dorsal fin that hides in crevasses during the day. 6-12 inches.

Queen Parrotfish (*Scarus vetula*) is a bright blue parrot with dramatic markings around the face and mouth. 12-18 inches.

Queen Triggerfish (*Balistes vetula*) is a striking, multi-hued flattish fish with striking facial markings and extended fin and tail tips. 8-16 inches.

Sharksucker (*Echeneis naucrates*) is a remora that attaches its disc to turtles, boat bottoms, sharks, and sometimes divers. They are harmless and can be pulled off easily. 10-18 inches.

Yellowhead Jawfish (*Opistognathus aurifrons*) is a thin pale fish that hovers above a hole into which it retreats tail-first if approached. Eggs are incubated within the mouth of the male. 2-3 inches.

EELS, SHARKS, AND RAYS (partial list of my favorites)

Spotted Moray (*Gymnothorax moringa*) is a large-bodied eel, heavily spotted with black on a pale underbody.

Goldentail Moray (*Gymnothorax miliaris*) is a spotted eel of gold, black, and brown.

Brown Garden Eel (*Heteroconger longissimus*) is a shy, small eel that lives in groups. En masse, they wave gracefully from their holes, catching plankton.

Nurse Shark (*Ginglymostoma cirratum*) is probably the only shark you will see. It lies docilely on the bottom or under rock ledges, where it should be left undisturbed.

Southern Stingray (*Dasyatis americana*) is a common ray that swims freely or lies on the bottom, often with only its eyes sticking out of the sand.

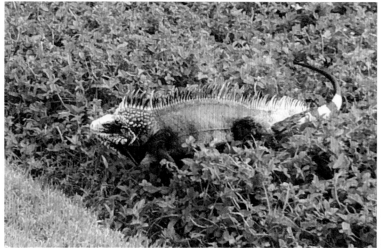

A Friendly Iguana.

Dianna Emory

Spotted Eagle Ray (*Aetobatus narinari*) is a large and lovely spotted ray with a pronounced head and snout.

REPTILES

Green Sea Turtles (*Chelonia mydas*), which are the most common turtle in the USVI, are only green on the inside where their fat lies. They have only two plates between their eyes, distinguishing them from the loggerheads that have two pairs. 3-4 feet; 250-450 pounds.

Hawksbill Sea Turtles (*Eretmochelys imbricata*) are common on Caribbean reefs. They are the only turtles with shell plates that overlap and are also distinguished by their overbite and serrated rear shell plates. 2.5-3 feet; 95-165 pounds.

Leatherback Sea Turtles (*Dermochelys coriacea*), pelagic turtles that feed on jellyfish, are the largest turtles. Their shells are covered with dark, leather-like skin, and they have no shell plates. 4-5.5 feet; 250-450 pounds.

Loggerhead Sea Turtles (*Caretta caretta*), with their large heads, are common on the Florida coast, but are rare in the USVI. One has nested on St. Croix. 2.5-3.5 feet; 155-375 pounds.

CORALS (partial list)

Elkhorn Coral (*Acropora palmata*)

Giant Brain Coral (*Colpophyllia natans*)

Staghorn Coral (*Acropora cervicornis*)

CRUSTACEANS AND GORGONIANS (partial list)

Spiny Lobster (*Panulirus argus*)

Common Sea Fan (*Gorgonia ventalina*)

Sea Rod (*Plexaura flexuosa*)

FLORA OF VIRGIN ISLANDS NATIONAL PARK[67, 68, 69, 70, 71, 72]

Virgin Islands National Park explodes with flowers, of which there are 740 species on the island of St. John. The following group of my favorites includes not only those that are native to the island but also those that are frequently used as ornamentals in local gardens, such as hibiscus. You will see that some of these plants are considered invasive by the Virgin Islands Department of Agriculture, Forestry Division. They are included for their appeal to pollinators and for your identification so that you can help to eradicate them. Latin names are provided first for flora to encourage us to stretch our minds and think in Latin.

FLOWERING PLANTS AND SHRUBS OF VIRGIN ISLANDS NATIONAL PARK (partial list)

Acalypha hispida (Chenille Plant/Monkey Tail) is a medicinal shrub with long pendulous chenille-like red "tails" comprised of many staminate flowers.

Antigonon leptopus (Mexican Creeper/Coral Vine) is an invasive that clambers over the hills and roadsides, often covering other vegetation with a plethora of small pink heart-shaped flowers. They are coveted by bees and wasps.

Anthurium andraeanum (Flamingo Flower), a member of the same family as the calla lily, typically boasts a waxy pink or red heart-shaped spathe. This dwarfs its barely noticeable real flower.

Asclepias curassavica (Tropical Milkweed), an evergreen perennial sub-shrub, attracts many pollinators, including monarch, painted lady, and swallowtail butterflies, wasps, and hummingbirds. A favorite plant for monarch egg-laying, its silky-haired seeds float from place to place on air currents.

Allamanda carhartica (Golden Trumpet/Buttercup Flower), which is often used as a cathartic, has large yellow tubular flowers growing on shrubs or sprawling vines.

Bougainvillea glabra (Paper Flower) sports profusely blooming bracts of red, pink, magenta, orange or white, which surround small white flowers.

Comocladia dodonaea (Christmas Bush) is a relative of poison ivy that can produce a burning rash. I am including this because of a personal and unpleasant encounter!

Datura candida (Angel's Trumpet/Angel's Tears), with its large and lovely white trumpet flowers and velvety bluish leaves, is extremely poisonous, containing a deadly psychoactive alkaloid (belladonna, henbane, mandrake).

Helliconia (Wild Banana) represents forty+/- species featuring brightly colored bracts, including *Helliconia tortuosa* that "recognize certain hummingbirds by the way the birds sip the flowers' nectar. The plants respond by allowing pollen to germinate, ultimately increasing the chances for successful seed formation"…"to our knowledge these findings provide the first evidence of pollinator recognition in plants," wrote the authors of a 2015 Oregon State University College of Forestry study.

Hibiscus schizopetalus (Coral Hibiscus/Fringed Hibiscus) produces a dainty little flower and is related to the more dramatic large-blossomed hibiscus hybrids. Buds picked from the shrub the night before will open the next morning and last for one day.

Lantana camara (Lantana) is a shrub with small, densely packed pink flowers producing impressive displays that attract pollinators.

Nerium oleander (Oleander), a profusely blooming poisonous pink shrub, can be kept bushy or allowed to grow up to twenty feet tall.

ORCHIDS (partial list)

Plumbago capensis (South African Leadwort) is a magnificent low-growing, pale blue-flowered shrub which flowers for most of the year.

Stephanotis floribunda (Madagascar Jasmine), a vine from the milk-weed family, produces very fragrant clusters of white-lobed flowers.

Thunbergia grandiflora (Sky Flower) produces yellow-throated, trumpet-shaped blue flowers that brighten roadsides and dry areas.

CACTI AND SUCCULENTS (partial list)

Acacia westiana (Sucker Cactus) is a prickly ground cactus that is quite annoying to hikers.

Agave americana (Century Plant), which likely originated in Mexico, is so-named because it seems to take a century to flower.

Aloe vera (Aloe/First Aid Plant) is a treatment for wounds, sunburn, and rashes.

Cephalocereus (Pipe Organ Cactus/Dildo Cactus) is often used by nest-building birds for protection from predators and strengthening of the nest.

Cereus (Columnar Cactus) is a yellow-centered white cactus that blooms at night on the Lind Point Trail.

Echinocactus grusonii (Barrel Cactus/Turk's Head) produces edible pink fruits and grows in formidable rocky areas.

Optunia ficus-indica (Paddle Cactus/Prickly Pear), with spines removed, are used in soup, salads, and desserts.

Optunia repens (Sucker Cactus) is a heavily-spined, low-growing cactus.

TREES OF VIRGIN ISLANDS NATIONAL PARK (partial list)

Virgin Islands National Park is home to more than 400 species of trees, many of which can be seen from the hiking trails, along the seashore, and at ruin sites.

*Native tree found in VINP

**Nonnative tree found in VINP (according to VINP)

***Invasive species, according to VINP Department of Agriculture, Forestry Division, as a result of a study funded through the USDA Forest Service. U.S. Executive order 131112 defines invasive species as "alien species whose introduction does or is likely to cause economic or environmental harm or harm to human health."

*Annona muricata** (Sugar Apple, Soursop), which produces round, sweet edible fruit with cancer-fighting properties, can be found in many locations on St. John.

*Bursera simaruba** (Gumbo Limbo/Turpentine) is a medicinal, dry forest tree which is easily distinguished by its red peeling bark.

Cassia fistula (Golden Shower), examples of which are found at Caneel Bay, hosts stunning clusters of golden flowers.

*Coccothrinax alta** (Teyer Palm/Broom Palm) is a tall, slender palm and the only palm native to the Virgin Islands. Used in fish traps and baskets, it prefers moist habitats.

*Cocoloba uvifera** (Seagrape) is a common shoreline tree which sports clusters of edible purple fruits.

*Cordia sebestena** (Geranium Tree) is found at Caneel Bay.

*Crescentia cujete** (Calabash) displays leaves that grow the length of its primary branches. Its large, round fruit is used as ornamental bowls and rattles.

*Delonix regia*** (Flamboyant Tree/Royal Poinciana), although not native, can frequently be seen on St. John. With its brilliant reddish orange flowers and long ferny leaves, it creates quite a spectacle. Local musicians make use of its shak shak pods.

Guaiacum officinale* (Lignum Vitae), the tree of life, produces blue flowers and orange seed pods. It is a favored shade tree.

Jacaranda acutifolia (Fern Tree) is a blue-flowered tree with ferny leaves.

Ceiba pentandra** (Kapok/Silk Cotton Tree) is a deciduous tree with a distinctive buttressed root system. Growing 150 foot+/-, kapoks can found on the Lameshur and Reef Bay trails. Its flowers attract bats and morning bees. The Tainos believed that the tree's spirit would communicate when it was ready to be transformed into an island-hopping canoe. Life jackets and mattresses were once stuffed with its pod silk.

Hippomane mancinella* (Manchineel) is distinguished by its small oval leaves and small green, poisonous "apples." All parts of this tree are highly toxic and should be avoided.

Hura crepitans** (Monkey No Climb/Sand Box Tree) has noticeable spikes covering its bark. No monkey would climb it.

Mangifera indica** (Mango) produces a popular and well-known fruit as well as welcome shade.

Melicoccus bijugatus*** (Genip) is a large, deciduous shade tree with small, tart edible fruit and bumpy gray bark.

Morinda citrifolia* (Noni, Painkiller Plant), with its large oval leaves, can be found at the entrance to Trunk Bay. Its cream-colored fruit is considered medicinal.

Pimenta racemosa* (Bay Rum Tree) is a tall, smooth-barked medicinal tree which can be found near Cinnamon Bay's ruins.

Plumeria alba* (Frangipani) typically sports fragrant white flowers with yellow centers, although imported pink varieties also exist. Its smooth-barked, long slender leaves are eaten by the magnificent yellow, black, and orange frangipani caterpillar, which becomes the large brown sphinx moth.

Rhizophora mangle* (Mangrove) is found in abundance on St. John's shores, providing critical habitat for many species. Its arching, splayed roots are noticeable.

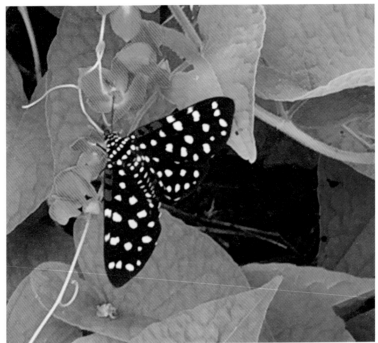

Dianna Emory

Invasive Mexican Creeper Feeds the Pollinators.

*Tamarindus indica*** (Tamarind) is a frequently-seen tree with lovely delicate leaves and 3-inch-long brown, tart fruits that look like seed pods. The fruit is used for beverages and preserves, as well as being a prime ingredient in Worcestershire sauce.

The related invasive, *Leucaena leucocephala* (Guinea Tamarind***), is the bane of local farmers. The guinea tamarind's merits rest in its value for erosion control and its protein-rich pods that provide feed for goats and cattle.

*Tecoma stans*** (Ginger Thomas) produces the lovely yellow trumpet-shaped flowers renowned as the official flower of the U.S. Virgin Islands. This nonnative tree is also noted for its long seedpods.

*Thespesia populnea*** (Maho) is found on the shoreline of its name-sake, Maho Bay. Heart-shaped leaves, seedpods, and pale yellow to purple flowers are its trademarks.

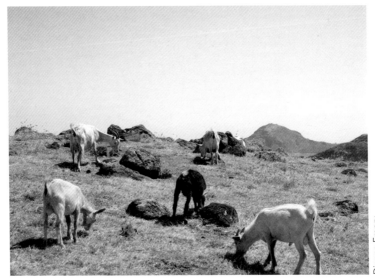

Dianna Emory

Island Goats.

THE THREAT OF INVASIVES
AND EXOTIC SPECIES

The Virgin Islands Department of Agriculture, Forestry Division, stresses the devastating impact of exotic invasive species. While non-threatening native species can grow in one part of the world and cause no harm, their effects "can harm native organisms directly by eating them, smothering them, or indirectly, by out-competing them for natural resources and crowding them out."[71] Animals like goats and pigs can be agriculturally beneficial but extremely destructive when roaming in the wild. Rats and mongoose are responsible for the depletion and extinction of many species of birds, reptiles, amphibians, invertebrates, and plants.

9

FROM YOUR NURTURING SPACE
TO YOUR OWN BACKYARD

*"My recollections of a hundred lovely lakes has given me blessed relief
from care and worry and the troubled thinking of the modern day.
It has been a return to the primitive and the peaceful."*
Hamlin Garland

Carefully examining two of our national parks and looking at the
other types of green spaces that are available can inspire us to seek
out more opportunities for involvement with the natural world. There
are so many conserved areas and green spaces just waiting for exploration, athletic engagement, and quiet contemplation. If we lived out our
days forever healthy, with no limitations on our ability to reach out to
those places, most of us would be quite happy. The reality is that there
are periods in nearly any person's life when we just can't take advantage
of all that nature holds. For those times, and for old age, we can find
comfort and our nature fix in our immediate environment. We can
immerse ourselves in elements of the natural world and supplement our
lack of access to grand adventures by making our environment greener
and deliberately bringing more living things into our life space.

CREATING YOUR SPACE

Bringing nature into your home does not need to mean finding a leathery squished squirrel on the wall behind your sofa. Yes, it did happen.
Following several months away from home, we returned to a lingering
sweet odor but could not find the source. All had been scrubbed repeatedly, and we just could not figure it out. Gradually, the odor dissipated
and we forgot about it—until we rearranged the furniture, pulled out
the sofa, and found the paper-thin squirrel corpse stuck to the wall.
The combination was deadly: children prone to leaving the deck door
open; a healthy population of gray squirrels anxious to find a handout;
and a son who routinely ran across the room, leaping onto the sofa, and
slamming it against the wall.

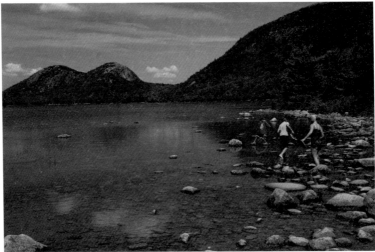

Sheridan Steele

Natural Stepping Stones for Fun Outdoors.

Physicians, architects, mental health professionals, nature enthusiasts, scientists, athletes, promoters of parks and green spaces, conservationists, and so many others—we are all trying to get people back out
into the green world to rediscover what we are threatened with losing;
to bring our bodies to their maximum level of fitness; and to place a
high value on this extraordinary place and its creatures. When we are
able, we get outdoors at every opportunity. We bring the outdoors close
to us as we place windows where we can see the details of the woods,
the fields, the waters, and the wildlife. We flock to community gardens,
the areas around our homes, parks, and other green spaces to inhale all
that they hold. When it is dark and cold or we are under the weather
ourselves, we watch lovely videos of the world and her creatures. And,
many of us build a living indoor space where we can derive some extra
pleasure from greenery with the knowledge that our plants are cleaning
the air as well.

A new biophilic architecture and design movement is intent on
altering interior spaces and cities so that interaction with nature happens routinely. Recognizing the impact of the natural world on well-
being and inspired by E.O. Wilson's concept of biophilia, "humankind's

natural affinity for life and its tendency to bond us with other living things," urban planners have a vision of cities within nature. For
instance, Singapore, once known as "A Garden City," now uses the
motto "A City in a Garden." The image is quite different. *Biophilic
Cities* author Timothy Beatley states that this increased connection
with the natural world is "all framed by the emerging research showing
nature's ability to make us healthier and happier."[6]

Let's begin by making a list of some of the things that we might
do to create a small nurturing space. When we choose, we can build it
out from there to include more of our interior environment. First, find
the space in your home. Mine is a north-facing window overlooking
our fields, sloping down to Eastern Bay. From here I can watch the
deer leaping and racing about in the field, assorted birds and squirrels
picking apples off a thirty-foot tree, and the condition of the surface
of the water for expeditions. A good comfortable chair is an important
element. Okay, that is there. Comfy. The next thing, from my perspective, are some houseplants with which I can build relationships. Those
plants really thrive when they are in a relationship, you know. From
within my current nurturing space, I am going to choose some that you
might love, too:

1) A large green-hued copper urn from Ben's mother's house,
   filled with an assortment of begonias—including foliosa,
   escargot, and pearcei—that came to me as babies from my
   friend, Annie. The container and the plants remind me of
   people I love.

2) Three phalaenopsis orchids, combinations of burgundy and
   white, which I gave myself. They remind me of my friend,
   Ruth Marie, who is also an orchid-lover.

3) One frilly, burgundy African violet, in a copper saucer that
   belonged to my mother. The violet is now large, but arrived in
   a tiny pot from my friend, Diana, many years ago.

4) Three blue streptocarpus from a birthday party Ben gave for
   me several years ago. I hope to keep them going as long as I
   keep going.

5) One rosary vine that is a relative of one that my grandmother

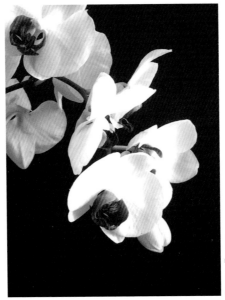

Have a Relationship with an Orchid.

gave me well over forty years ago. Gifts of my rosary's babies have gone to many friends and family members.

Next, I need a terrarium. Fortunately, since it is still winter, I already have one. It is large and wrought iron and was hauled from the basement of the Smithsonian by Dr. W. C. Kendall for his little girl, my grandmother Minerva. She kept it for much of her life, then turned it over to me when I was in the throes of my PTSD pre-adolescence. That aquarium/terrarium has since housed everything from tropical fish to newts and lake trout to baby snakes, turtles, and a host of plants. It now is filled with only plants, special rocks, lichens, mosses, and some attractive sticks. It rests in its retirement years in our living room with one corner rusting away. I think you can see the importance of history in your nurturing space. Do you have some containers or plants with a history? What other elements do you want to include there? They don't all need to be plants and containers. Maybe a source of music or a special view? Oh, my Foxy Kitty has climbed into the chair, thus she is now at least a temporary part of my space. Ben's space. His chair! Our space. Your turn. Tell me about your nurturing space over the miles and how you will build out from it so that your entire home feels nurturing, inside and out.

PLAYING WITH PLANTS
"Spare time in the garden, either digging, setting out, or weeding; there is no better way to preserve your health."
English Gardener, 1699

El plans for the future—a time when she is sure she will be healthier. She carefully sketches out the details of additions to her garden, indicating where she wants each shrub, tree, and plant to go. She visualizes her completed garden in her mind's eye and then paints lovely watercolors of what she sees. When she has trouble sleeping or is in pain, she focuses on all that her garden will hold. Colors may be vibrant or subtle, forms may be spikey or graceful, and paths can wind invitingly around a corner or take one directly toward a special piece of sculpture. She envisions the bees and butterflies that will flit amongst the blossoms, going deep into the patterns on their wings and bodies. She watches a small green frog climb upon a lily pad and then hop off into the cool water of her pool. And, when she brings herself back to her fully alert state, she feels much better in every way. Suddenly, two exciting thoughts pop into her mind. She will save her watercolors to give to her friends, rather than leaving them in her files. And, she will ask the library if they would like her to develop a landscaping plan for them.

Ed and Sharon are at a point in life, with two young children and busy careers, where they don't have much time on their own. Here in the Northeast, it is dark for many months both in the morning when they head for work and at night when they get home. To satisfy some of their need for green space, with their children they grow bulbs and seedlings along with their houseplants, creating a plethora of exploding growth that cleans toxins from the air while providing a green oasis within their home. Even kitty has a part in this as she chews upon the flat of grass and catmint that is grown for her pleasure. As the days lengthen and the soil warms, seedlings are moved into the outdoor beds to receive family nurturing as they grow to produce edible delights and armloads of bouquets, many of which are delivered to area nursing homes.

Frank, on the other hand, loves the rototilling and soil preparation that will provide what his vegetable garden and dahlias need to produce spectacularly. His lung cancer has slowed him down a bit, but through it all, his garden has provided the opportunity for investment of mind and body that he feels have kept him going.

Rita appears at each horticultural exhibit with award-winning blooms. She is so personally invested in the production of these glorious specimens that she finds herself focusing on their care even while she receives her chemotherapy. She jokes that soon she will begin growing hair as well as she grows flowers.

Andy is angry at his cancer and feels like physically attacking the illness. He yanks the weeds away from the many gardens he tends as if they were the cancer cells. He stomps on them from time to time or rips them into shreds. When he puts them in the composter he delights in transforming them from weeds to healthy soil. Andy's treatment of the weeds is ripe for incorporation into the visualization training that will focus on eradicating cancer cells.

Ethel, a spritely ninety-year-old breast cancer survivor, tells me that her African violets, gloxinia, and other houseplants help her to look forward to each day. She has nurtured many of them for years, in the same way that she has cared for her own body since her diagnosis decades ago. Although she has had recurrences of cancer over the years, and many related surgeries, she is currently healthy and sparkling with energy. She cares for every plant as one would a child—feeding, pruning, and bathing each one religiously and carefully repotting them when they outgrow their space. One of her greatest joys comes from dividing her plants and passing the offspring on to friends and lonely nursing home patients.

How satisfying it is to dig deep into that rich, dark earth, crumbling the soil in one's hands, hollowing out a cozy nest for a tiny seedling, and then gently patting the dirt into place so it will support the little plant as it grows. The process of preparing the soil to receive seeds and young plants has captured the hearts of many. Or, how about sticking some unpromising-looking brown bulbs into a pot or a patch of soil, with the knowledge that months later they will be bursting into bloom? For others, the greatest satisfaction comes from the weeding out of intruders, the pinching back or pruning to strengthen the plant, or the deadheading to encourage repeat blooms. Whether attacking the weeds and burning off some tension or doing the nurturing tasks of planting, pinching, pruning, and deadheading, the mental health benefits abound. There are also those gardeners who derive the most pleasure from the production of show-quality specimens or prolific bouquets and others who stimulate their brains through learning the Latin names of their plants, incorporating as many Latin challenges as possible into their gardens.

Sometimes it is the process of building the garden as a part of a landscaping plan that captivates or the satisfaction of strolling among the plants inhaling their fragrance and delighting in their beauty that addicts us to gardening. And, there are those among us who view their garden plots and plants as a way to host others—from people to birds, bees, bugs, and animals—or as an opportunity to produce healthy food. Whatever the source of the pleasures we derive from our horticultural interests—whether they focus on acres of carefully landscaped gardens or a few herbs on a windowsill—this great national obsession also has enormous potential to assist us when we are in a crisis.

The satisfaction, pride, and fulfillment that come from tending plants are terrific stress-reducers. Let's go indoors for a moment to your orchid, African violet, or streptocarpus. If you are an avid gardener, you don't need me to tell you about the relationships that can be built with plants. Many of our plants can live for years, giving us a touchstone with another being as we move through the peaks and valleys of life. Earlier, I mentioned some of my favorite plants, each of which I will tell you a bit more about. As I look toward my huge pot of three varieties of begonias, my mind drifts to my friend Annie Judd who years ago produced miniature versions of these plants for each of our Garden Club of Mount Desert members as a part of a horticultural challenge. Annie, a great horticulturalist and inspirational gardener, nurtures her plants from seeds and cuttings, passing many along to her grateful pals. Her little begonias joined one another in a huge brass pot to live happily together and produce great pleasure as they have grown and bloomed, triggering thoughts of Annie each time I look at them. Those thoughts also include the award-winning Charlotte Rhoades Butterfly Garden, in Southwest Harbor, Maine, that Annie resurrected. There she raises and releases hundreds of threatened monarch butterflies each year. Back in my indoor garden, there is the burgundy African violet, given to me by Diana Wister, one of the most generous-spirited and spiritual women I have ever known. She reaches out in every direction, bestowing kindness to all. Now ten years old, Diana's violet keeps blooming and blooming beside its graceful streptocarpus friend, a table centerpiece from a birthday party Ben threw for me several years ago. There is one more important indoor plant I must mention again. That is the rosary plant that my grandmother, Nanny Minerva, gave me over forty years ago. Nanny lives on in that plant as I snip and root cuttings, passing them on to cherished friends when they are as well-established as the friendships. I think you know where I am going with all of this talk of individual plants and the relationships we have with them. As much as you and I love getting out there and taking the challenge of dividing a tap-rooted baptisia to establish its offspring, hauling a huge rhododendron across the yard on a tarp to its new home, or shoveling truckloads of soil into place, there is much satisfaction to be gained from any connection with the greenness of plants, even if we are at the point where it is a challenge just to pick up the watering pitcher.

Do you have some favorite houseplants, garden plants, or gardening jobs? You might want to jot them down, along with any aspirations to expand your projects. Or, if you are new to indoor and outdoor gardening, we will consider where you can begin. There is a great green world out there full of many opportunities for discovery that can begin with your own increasingly green thumb.

There is much evidence out there in the world of research studies that gardening keeps our minds and our bodies fit and healthy. That goes for indoor as well as outdoor plant activities, thus we have the opportunity to derive great benefits from gardening regardless of what life challenges we are facing. There is nothing new about this premise, which dates back two thousand years to Taoists who looked to the creation and enjoyment of gardens as routes to good health. In 1792, William Tuke encouraged psychiatric patients to work in the gardens of asylums and care for the animals there in an attempt to focus their attentions on external activities. "This nonpunitive treatment system, emphasizing acceptance and the natural surroundings of a living environment, formed the basis of humane treatment standards which are still applicable (in hospitals) today."[33] Centuries later, the "eye pastures" that could be seen from indoors at mental health hospitals in the early 1900's paved the way toward using gardening as a treatment for post-traumatic stress disorder.

A Texas A&M researcher, Roger Ulrich, provided reassurance that "simply enjoying a patch of green, even from afar, can be therapeutic." When comparing "hospital records from patients recovering from

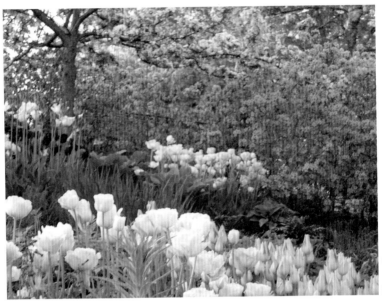

Dianna Emory

The Miracle of Bulbs and Spring's Rebirth.

gallbladder surgery, he discovered that the ones whose rooms had a view of nature recovered more quickly than those who looked out at a brick wall."[34]

Several studies have demonstrated that gardening may lower the risk for dementia and numerous others have shown that gardeners are more likely to be compassionate, reaching out to try and help others, and that their social relationships are more advanced, according to Fran Sorin, author of *Digging Deep: Unearthing Your Creative Roots through Gardening*.[35] We also know that gardening allows each of us to be a nurturer and that those without close family and friends can find great rewards in building relationships with their plants, in the same manner that they do with their pets.

Another report tells us that we eat less when we are gardening and burn an average of 265 calories an hour, more than expended by brisk walking. If you are like me, wrapped from head to toe in a screened bug suit that will not allow the ticks, black flies, or mosquitoes inside, and you are also covered with mud, the reason for not reaching for a snack (or even lunch) relates to having to extricate oneself from the outfit and go indoors. Sticking your water bottle up under the suit without trapping one of the clouds of flying insects is enough of a challenge. And then there is the need to duck into the bushes which holds a few surprises of its own, like a tick in the wrong place. Yes, it happened.

Hauling soil, shoveling, or lifting rocks for walls for 30 minutes or more can build up more than just a healthy sweat—five days a week of this can increase your metabolic rate threefold to fivefold according to the University of South Carolina's Dr. Steven Blair,[36] thus reducing blood pressure and improving cholesterol levels. Any activity that is strenuous enough to make you slightly winded improves your cardiovascular fitness. Even reaching to prune a vine or carrying a pitcher to water those indoor plants can help your body to maintain a level of fitness. As you engage in gardening, positive emotions can grow along with your plants as you relax and let go, exercise at whatever level is comfortable for you, and cruise into the zone of altered consciousness that is induced through many repetitive activities, including meditation.

Our horticultural indulgences hold great rewards for us when we are working our way through illness, crisis, or regular life. With their assistance, we can move ourselves forward into a healthier space.

THE CREATURE CONNECTION

An elderly Alzheimer's patient sits staring out his window, giving no sign of recognition when his visitors and nurse enter the room. Not, that is, until he hears a sharp yelp, spins around, and opens his arms to the retriever puppy darting toward him. "Oh, good dog," he says, "how I've missed you."

Nine-year-old Mary lies amidst the fresh golden shavings on the stall floor, her head nestled in the crook of her big bay gelding's jaw and throat. Ranger is spread out across the stall, snuffling gently. This position seems to be a comforting one for Mary, who feels so at home with the horses, as she contemplates the loss of her father.

I bury my face in the soft brown fur of our old coon cat's coat. The tears run down my face onto Mickey's head as he purrs loudly and rubs his face against mine. Somehow he knows that I am sad and need his love now more than ever.

A cerebral-palsied child is hoisted upon a solid gray mare as her expression is transformed from resignation to joy. She is secured on the saddle as she bends down to place her face affectionately on her horse's mane, then off she goes down the polo cross field at a full gallop. This child, who just moments ago has been slumped in a wheelchair, is now sticking to her saddle like a little tick as her mount takes her not only to the end of the field, but also to elation.

Frankie has spent most of his six years of life in the institution that is his home. After years of almost no communication with humans, other than to occasionally roll a ball back in his therapist's direction, we are having a breakthrough. He looks directly at me, stares down at the dwarf black and white rabbit in my lap, reaches out, and puts his hand on her. This bunny will be Frankie's bridge to playing outdoors and to communication with people, great strides forward for a little autistic boy who has spent the bulk of every day for several years rubbing the same spot on the wall.

These life snapshots and multitudes more illustrate the important role that animals play in our lives. Acceptance, love, tactile stimulation, eagerness, and a touchstone with reality are offered up unconditionally by our dogs, cats, horses, goats, and the rest of the animals. Some fish, a turtle, or a parakeet can give us a reason to get up every day, care for another living thing and move forward in what may sometimes seem an overwhelming life. If you are thinking that fish don't live very long, you might be interested to know that the oldest reported goldfish to have lived in a bowl passed away at age 43. If I got a goldfish today, he or she could surely outlive me.

History and research support the importance of pets in our lives. The interrelationship of humans and animals has existed since recorded history, with the employment of pets as psychotherapeutic adjuncts dating back to the early Egyptians, who designated cats as deities connected to the sun god. Over the centuries, other beliefs developed about pets and their impact on humans. Dogs in ancient Babylon were portrayed as the companions of Gula, the god of healing, and "the tongue of a dog" was prescribed as a remedy for low spirits. Kelly states, "Ever since humans domesticated wild dogs some 14,000 years ago, the bond between people and their animals has been a remarkable mix of need and affection, practicality and indulgence. Begun when the two species discovered that hunting cooperatively was more beneficial than competing, that early alliance has taught a lesson that is still being studied today: health benefits—indeed survival—could result from having a pet."[21] Equine-related therapy had its beginnings in ancient Greece, where the chronically pain-ridden were sent to the gymnasiums to ride selected horses on cross-country outings.[22] Priests theorized that these jaunts would lighten their patients' moods and provide respite from pain. We would view this alliance as the intersection of nature and her creatures. This reminds me of an old friend whose physician suggested she begin riding with me to help ease her chronic back pain. Timid at first, Penny became a proficient rider whose back responded well to her time on a horse. Her spirits were lifted as well as we rode through the surrounding beauties of our national park, encountering various wild creatures along the way.

The Delta Society was founded in the United States in 1977 for the purpose of bringing together individuals who were interested in pursuing the connection of people, animals, and the environment. In the same year, the first facility dedicated to the study of social and psychological relationships between people and animals, The Center on Interaction of Animals and Society, was established at the University of Pennsylvania. Later, the pet/owner bond was the subject of a 1979 conference at the University of Dundee.

Friedman and Katcher[23] postulated that pets provide seven functions, each of which benefits human health. These include something to care for, touch, and keep one busy; companionship, which has the capacity to both reduce the frequency of serious disease and prolong life; focus of attention, which draws one away from distressing thoughts; safety, which decreases depression and is likely to have direct psychological and physiological health benefits; and exercise that promotes both physical health and social interaction. Levinson[24] reported the therapeutic benefits of pet-facilitated therapy for adults and children in outpatient and inpatient settings. In describing the use of animals for emotionally disturbed, deaf, blind, and/or developmentally-delayed children, he proposed that pets act as transitional objects with the child first forming a relationship with the pet, then with the therapist, and, finally, with others. Katcher determined that keeping animals which one talked to and petted produced feelings "of reverie and comfort"[25] and enhanced longevity and physical health. In their work with post-coronary patients, Beck and Katcher[26] concluded that the survival rate of those patients who had a pet to care for was statistically greater than those who did not have a pet.

Specific to the elderly, Riddick[27] explored the impact of aquariums on elderly subsidized housing residents. Those introduced to aquariums as a hobby demonstrated significant changes in their relaxation states, diastolic blood pressure, and overall leisure satisfaction. Alzheimer's patients isolated by their disease were found to improve in their social interaction when pets were used as catalysts.[28] In a study of depressed and medically ill outpatients, McCulloch[29] looked at the impact of pets on loneliness, isolation, activity level, morale, sense of humor, and

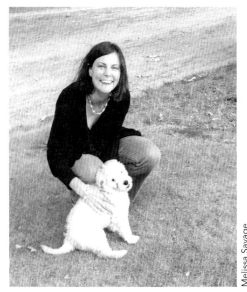

A Puppy Can Make a Difference.

other factors. Regardless of whether the pet belonged to the subject or someone else in the household, the impact of the pet improved general mood, according to two-thirds of the patients. Studies of retirees living alone yielded interesting results for those given parakeets versus those given houseplants to care for, concluding five months later that all of those with parakeets exhibited enhanced communication and contact with other people, compared to plants.[30] In a hospital setting, Corson and Corson worked with psychiatric patients who were described as uncommunicative, withdrawn, and self-centered. With the introduction of pet therapy, they described a "widening circle of warmth"[31] that began with tactile and non-verbal communication with the animal and progressed to include other patients, therapists, and staff.

Because of the attention that animals require, they can build a bridge back into nature and the outdoors for us. And, at times, they may be the one hands-on contact we have with the natural world. No wonder we spend thousands on their care, treat them as our children

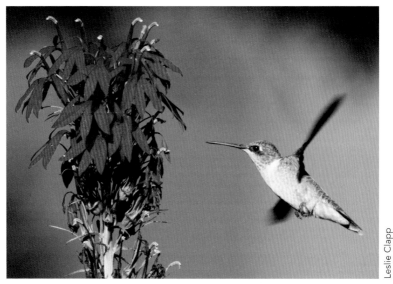

Leslie Clapp

Ruby-throated Hummingbird on Cardinal Flower.

and partners, give them as gifts to those we love, and mourn their deaths so grievously.

When we or our loved ones move into old age or face crises, the pets in our lives can become even more important. Spending time with them, stroking their coats, giving them walks and treats, dedicating some of every day to their care, and talking to them when we just cannot verbalize our fears and pain to our human companions can make all the difference.

Like our companion animals, creatures in the wild give us additional comfort and stimulation. How thrilling it is to see an animal while exploring the outdoors. We grab our cameras, hoping to record the sighting and then happily share it by email or on Facebook. Can you think of times when you have spotted an animal or bird that was particularly exciting and how quickly you wanted to share the experience with someone else? One fine day while biking in Everglades National Park, I rounded a corner and was astounded to see a Florida panther passing directly in front of me, only ten feet away. With a tawny flash

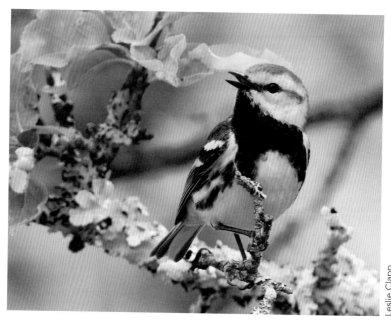

Leslie Clapp

Black-throated Green Warbler Travels from Maine to the Caribbean.

he was gone, but he has never disappeared from my visual memory. We reported that sighting to the park superintendent, as it is a rare thing to see a panther. That visit to the Everglades brought many other rewarding sightings of bobcats, alligators, crocodiles, and the most magnificent birds. A trip hiking in the desert mountains of Arizona's Saguaro National Park rewarded us with a close-up view of a gila monster; Grand Teton presented moose, bear, and elk; and Acadia has given us scores of animal sightings. Within Northeastern communities, among others we see coyotes, woodchucks, skunks, foxes, raccoons, deer, and the occasional moose or bear. We really do live with the animals.

How glorious it is to wake to the sound of birdsongs outside one's window. Right now, can you think of a particular bird's call and get an auditory sense of how it sounds? The hermit thrush, the wood thrush, the robin, and the chickadee alert our auditory senses as we delight in their songs. Even the caw of a crow or the raspy voice of a raven draws one into nature. Birding has become one of the most popular outdoor activities, particularly for seniors. Whether on outdoor expeditions or from within our own homes, we derive great pleasure and intellectual stimulation from bird watching. As we do for our companion animals, we can really spend the dollars on those birds between seeds and suet, birdhouses and birdbaths, and feeders of every variety, none of which is truly squirrel-proof. But, they surely pay us back in the joy they deliver. As we age, studying the details of different bird species, learning their calls, and discovering how to identify them in flight or on our feeders presents hours of intellectual challenge that can help to keep our brains sharp. One birdsong expert recommends getting acquainted with birds and their songs in the same way you do people—looking at them as individuals with defining characteristics. He also suggests improving one's auditory memory through recording birdsongs and sketching out the song patterns.[32] If you strive to learn more about birds, good places to start are local, state, and National Audubon, Cornell Lab of Ornithology, and the apps, iBird Pro, EBird, and Audubon Bird.

10

VOLUNTEERISM IMPROVES
YOUR QUALITY OF LIFE

"To cherish what remains of the Earth and to foster its renewal
is our only legitimate hope of survival."
Wendell Berry

We sat one January day overlooking the turquoise waters of the Virgin Islands with our wise conservationist friend whose family generosity gave roots to this part of the National Park System. In his own right, Larry is dedicated to land conservation, volunteering on behalf of that and other important causes. Ben and I talked with him about how each of us can make some kind of a difference in this challenged world. His advice is well worth sharing. "Find your niche," he began. That really sums it up, for your niche and your passion can carry you a very long way as you work to assist an important project. Finding your niche is not so hard if you begin by thinking about what aspect of our world excites you the most and then how your areas of expertise and interest can be of benefit to a particular cause.

Can you reflect on some focus areas that inspire your passion? Now list your skill set and the kinds of activities with which you could assist. If you know of nonprofits that cater to the causes that interest you, make note of them or check out the Internet. Then think about what you would like to do for them if you could choose. Each of us has a skill set that can be very helpful to the causes we care about. Depending upon what else is going on in our lives, we may elect to engage deeply at some times and only a few hours a month at other times. The nonprofits that you approach might ask you to help them in ways that you had not considered, opening up a new adventure for you. Most nonprofits are enthusiastic about donated expertise and energy. Particularly during challenging times, what we can give of ourselves to others can help us to feel better about our own life circumstances.

Let's now expand on the concept of volunteerism and the ways it can enrich your life experience. Here is a story of how I got there and how a friend who took the time to advise me saved my daughter's life...

A Tribute to Richard Rockefeller

The path toward volunteerism was laid early for me as I struggled through an aggressive childhood cancer. Gratefully spared but anxious, I begged to be around for each next birthday over the first 12 years or so of life. A touchstone was provided by my grandmother, one of Washington, D.C.'s early environmental stewards, whose own ichthyologist and physician father had offered her the same. Together we recycled, counted returning migrating birds, and examined the summer shores of Sebago Lake for hints of overuse damages as she brought me out of myself. The message was clear: You are a part of the world community. Don't waste your precious days. Identify your passion, and do all that you can to make a difference in whatever gift of time you have.

Give or take 67 years later, I found myself not only alive but in a 400+ crowd at the Schoodic Institute in Winter Harbor, Maine. These conservation-minded people were hopeful that this science, research, and education nonprofit working on behalf of Acadia National Park and its abutting waters could bolster the economy of eastern Maine and assist Acadia, while also ferreting out and addressing major changes in our natural environment with its international conservation partners. As I looked around the crowd, I saw the faces of so many who had pursued their passions and given of mind, body, and spirit to a host of volunteer projects. From Friends of Acadia and Maine Coast Heritage Trust, where I have enjoyed volunteer leadership roles, to local hospital funders, art enthusiasts, national environmental and political leaders, they were clearly enriched through their histories of generosity. Their faces glowed with determination and their depth of dedication filled the room with something palpable.

As I listened to Secretary of the Interior Sally Jewell, Director of the National Park Service Jon Jarvis, and former Vice Chairman of the National Park Foundation Board, David Rockefeller, Jr., extoll the virtues of Schoodic Institute, and its potential impact on important environmental issues, I reflected back one year to the summer of 2013. A group of Maine Coast Heritage Trust supporters gazed from our terrace overlooking Eggemoggin Reach and its Acadia National Park-held easement islands. We talked about how volunteers before us had left a legacy to the Maine coast. We spoke of the need to inspire a new generation of stewards and to use our own time wisely. My husband, Ben, and I later acknowledged the power of change that lay within that handful of friends. Some worked on behalf of medical breakthroughs, others tirelessly counted birds while examining ecological mismatches, many engaged in land protection issues, and our physician friend, Richard Rockefeller, spent hundreds of volunteer hours fundraising for land conservation and, separately, exploring the depths of Post Traumatic Stress Disorder.

Richard is gone now, swept away in a tragic accident while headed on a volunteer mission. His spirit guides my pen, and his lessons steer me toward a commitment to work till my own end to see that his passions and Ben's and mine are further secured. For, you see, Richard's impact went well beyond his role as my friend and conservation mentor. I owe him a debt of gratitude for his important role in helping to save my daughter. When cancer snuck from behind and tried to snatch her away, he took the time to pull me aside. His advice changed the planned course of medical intervention and took her to an experimental clinical trial that is now standard treatment for similarly-threatened women. Generosity of spirit works in many ways.

In a fraction of a second, all can change. So, lend a helping hand, clean the roadside, make the call, or write the check: your opportunity is now. Together, we *can* make the difference. As you take the challenge, improve your own well-being, and rejoice in your good fortune at being a part of this place at this point in time. Instill in your heirs the spirit of giving back through creative energy, time, and dollars. Their own lives and the world will be richer for it.

This might be a good time for you to think more about your own strengths and passions. It may be that you are already investing a portion of each week in some volunteer effort, or perhaps you are searching for a place to give back. If you again think about what you care most about and how you would like to help things to move forward, there is a place for you. Over the years, your focus might change. For instance, in my early professional years when I was maintaining a busy practice in the mental health field and raising a young family, I was drawn to board work on behalf of our regional counseling center as well as to a school for emotionally and mentally challenged children. Now, my volunteer efforts are almost completely in the conservation and environmental arena—both of which also impact every person's mental health. A common thread always runs through.

If your thoughts turn to volunteering on behalf of our parks, conserved spaces, and the environment, you will find yourself useful regardless of the number of hours you can spare each week. And, your energy level can find a fit. From doing citizen science research to making phone calls to making fundraising visits, from stamping envelopes to shoveling snow—there is a job for you. You are guaranteed to feel that you have made a difference each time you put your time and energy to work. Where do you think that you can make a difference?

As you read and learn of threats to our natural world, you can also network with others and maintain contact with your congressional delegation—a way to reach beyond your own backyard to work on behalf of your cause. An example of one crisis relates to the impact of noise pollution on wildlife in protected areas. According to *The Wall Street Journal*, mating calls go unheard, fish are deafened, and animals are scared off as noise levels have been increased up to 10 decibels above natural levels.[73] Other crises in protected areas that you can express your feelings about include pollution of the night sky by excessive lighting, governmental threats to remove protection from some federal lands, and the recreational use of drones in conserved areas.

Perhaps your interests lead you to reach toward the domesticated and wild animals that have for years captivated you. Given how many of us connect with the creatures of our world, let's spend some time looking at how we can help them. There are many ways that we can give back to those beloved companion animals that give us the excuse to get outdoors, exercise, and feel better. They need us in order to eat, take care of their daily habits, and burn off their energy. Their wild cousins need us in other ways. One example relates to helping them out as they "synurbanize" and adapt to a changing world, according to *Northern Woodlands*.[74] This means paying attention to animal routes near roadways; avoiding poisons of any type and understanding how they travel through the food chain; and planting the green spaces around our homes to encourage wildlife.

Endless opportunities exist to give wild and companion animals the extra assistance they need to have a better quality of life or, in some cases, even survive. Forever etched in my mind is that first jolt into a sickening awareness of need on a frigid January day in eastern Maine. From the trash-heaped barnyard of a horse trader's farm, a dark rabbit warren of ramshackle corridors led into the depths of his barn. I caught a shadowy glimpse of the horses, goats, and other animals packed into the filthy stalls when an occasional shaft of light made it though the boarded windows. Far in the back, in the blackest space of all, was the gelding I had called about. "Dark's for the worms," the horse trader grumbled. "I keep worms in them stalls." He kept horses and goats, too. Dozens were scattered outside across the frozen fields, scrawny and shuddering in a strong northwest wind. Many were low-slung pregnant mares and nanny goats. Others, like the ones in the bowels of the barn, were shut away in that dark space for the winter with no reliable access to clean water, daylight, fresh bedding, or love. The horse trader shoved open the stall door, whipped a chain lead around a soft brown nose, and led us both out through the network of corridors and stalls, finally emerging into glaring sunlight and howling wind. Quivering and wild-eyed, matted with mud and manure, the scrawny young gelding danced and reared at the end of the lead line. "I'll take him," I muttered hastily, scrawling out numerals on a check, swallowing hard, and wishing I could buy and house the whole herd. A few months of careful nurturing produced a sleek, shiny bay coat, a loving disposition, and a gentle manner. Plump and fit, "Brownie" was passed on to a welcoming new home by summer's end. I fear that his barn mates were not so fortunate. The "need" screamed at me that day and has been echoed dozens of times since in media reports of animal abuses and rescues. We are regularly reminded of the desperate search for new homes for those animals and others whose owners can no longer keep them. You can help them and be rewarded many times over.

Each domesticated animal that we help can become a cherished family member; a partner for the lonely; a vehicle toward greater self esteem for a young caregiver; a source of humor and joy; a communication bridge for a depressed adolescent; an inspiration to an owner to get out and exercise; and a companion with whom the deepest feelings can be safely shared. Animal rescue and adoption holds the promise not only of improved life circumstances for needy animals but also of greatly enriched lives for the future owners. Jennifer Skiff, a dear friend who has produced two books, *The Divinity of Dogs* and *God Stories*, has dedicated her life to saving dogs internationally. My sister, Lois, a busy professional, somehow finds the time to help to arrange to transport truckloads of dogs shipped from southern states, foster them, and deliver them to their new homes. In the process, she has broadened her own relationship network.

To positively impact our environment and its creatures, we can also promote improved pet owner behavior, as suggested in a brochure that my daughter, Bethany Savage, and I put together for the SPCA of Hancock County (Maine). *Pets in Parks and on Preserves: Pet Etiquette Suggestions for Pets and Their Owners* focuses on how responsible owners can reduce the harm done to wildlife by companion animals. While on protected lands, dog owners can leash their dogs to prevent chasing, injury, and death of wildlife; disruption of nesting areas; intrusion into animal burrows and homes; and damage to rare and endangered plant life. Leashing also prevents unpleasant encounters with skunks and porcupines. Cleaning up after one's dogs is a thoughtful gesture to other people and the environment. Spay/neutering reduces the numbers of unattended and wandering dogs that chase and prey on wildlife and who do not receive proper care. Likewise, cat owners intending to reduce the feral cat and unwanted cat population through spay/neutering help to reduce decimation of the bird population; lower the threat to amphibians, reptiles, and small animals from roaming cats; and reduce the number of cats without adequate shelter and care. Recent statistics from Cornell Lab of Ornithology indicate that more than 2.4 billion birds are killed by cats each year in the United States.[75] Cat lovers who keep their pets indoors can protect wildlife and ensure the safety of their cats by protecting them from predators and vehicles. Conveying these messages takes time and energy. Your help could make a difference to the creatures of our world, both wild and domesticated.

Volunteering to help to get children's groups out into the natural world is another area where there is desperate need. Children can be enticed to spend more time outdoors due to their natural curiosity about and love of animals. Activities with animals often stimulate much greater interest for children than those where animals are not involved. Using connections with animals, whether dog walking or learning animal tracking, can provide an added incentive to young people to abandon their indoor toys in favor of nature. There is much data indicating that children and adults who regularly use the outdoors are healthier physically and emotionally. Likewise, a plethora of research exists related to the direct correlation between animal abuse and domestic violence and the transference of learned positive interaction with animals to appropriate interaction with humans.[76, 77]

Connecting kids and domesticated animals with a goal of positively impacting the environment, wildlife, and humans relates to the national movement to get children back outdoors for play and education. Richard Louv's landmark book, *Last Child in the Woods: Saving Our Children from Nature-Deficit Disorder*, launched an international effort to reconnect youth with nature. As Richard Louv states, " Children need nature for the healthy development of their senses, and, therefore, for learning and creativity. This need is revealed in two ways: by an examination of what happens to the senses of the young when they lose connection with nature; and by witnessing the sensory magic that occurs when young people—even those beyond childhood—are exposed to even the smallest direct experience of a natural setting."[77] Subsequent to Louv's work, the "No Child Left Inside" movement sought to promote environmental education for kindergarteners through twelfth graders. At Acadia National Park, former Superintendent Sheridan Steele made

Louv's initiative a primary part of his platform, effectively driving forward efforts on behalf of children and nature.

A similar effort aimed at getting kids outdoors while helping to protect creatures is the National Wildlife Federation and Disney Conservation Fund collaborative effort, the NWF Butterfly Heroes campaign, which encourages families to plant and care for native plants that support monarch butterflies. Protection of the monarchs runs to your own gardens, where you can plant Aesclepius (milkweed), a primary food of the monarch. If you are inclined to volunteer on behalf of pollinators, there are many other things you can plant to encourage them—monardas, echinaceas, salvias, and other flowers are especially tasty to pollinators, as are the dandelions and the clovers that grow on lawns. You might even consider striving to make your property a National Wildlife Federation Certified Wildlife Habitat. My friends, Leslie Clapp and Blaise DiSibour, have done a remarkable job with their property, making it a welcoming spot for all sorts of critters seeking native species. I will never reach the bar set by Leslie, president of Downeast Audubon, but it is fun trying. In addition to developing a wildlife-friendly yard that she opens to the public, she also produces a wide range of educational material related to birds and other wildlife through her volunteer work at Downeast Audubon.

Bringing children into the mix as you carve off a piece of your yard for native species helps to build a foundation of respect for the natural world that can last a lifetime. Encouraging children to get outdoors, while teaching them respect for other living things as they run and jump about, will lift the spirits and strengthen the bodies of the children and the volunteer.

There are so many valuable experiences out there just waiting for you. Once again, I cannot stress strongly enough how the engagement with others who need some help—whether people or causes—can bring you out of yourself to the point where you are deriving great benefit as well. Things just don't seem as overwhelming or hopeless in your own life when you can see that you are having some positive impact in the world. You likely have already conjured up many prospective places where your volunteer efforts could be of great use. If not, I am going to give you a

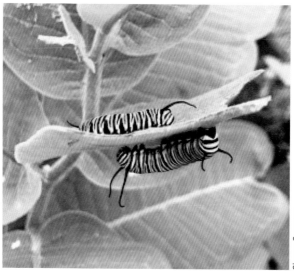

Sherry Streeter

Plant Milkweed for Monarchs.

few ideas that relate to the themes of this book. Before we get to that, how about a dose of laughter related to some stories of volunteerism?

Two distinguished elderly ladies, one the primary founder of Maine Coast Heritage Trust and numerous national causes, and the other a key figure at MOMA and the New York Botanical Garden, embark on a trip down east to examine a potential conservation project. Sensitive to their identities as wealthy summer folks from Mount Desert, they drive an unobtrusive Chevy with Maine plates down the long, snowy road. Soon hopelessly stuck and before the days of cell phones, they strike out to bare their identities in exchange for a good tow.

Bill, a generous-spirited retired physician turned fundraiser, embarks on one of his early fundraising visits equipped with his bag of materials that includes bios of the intended prey as well as detailed information about their giving history and numerous suggestions about how to approach them, complete with script. Driving away from the visit, he realizes that his bag has been left in the prospect's living room.

A major donor couple sits with the leader of a small nonprofit in anticipation of making another big gift, which has some contingencies. The president thanks them for their past generosity and then says, "Now that we've got that out of the way, I want to tell you I am really upset about the way you want to structure this gift." Hmmm. Did they make the gift? You guess.

Nervously perched on the edge of my chair in the Beverly Hills Four Seasons, I watch a parade of somewhat familiar-looking people streaming into the restaurant. I am not a TV viewer, as you will see. My host walks toward me, a man I have never met before and have cold-called from Maine, where I am board chair of Friends of Acadia. Dick Wolf joins me and remarks on his morning's interaction with various famous personalities. I remark on what must be the challenging nature of his show, *LA Law*. Bemused, he says, "Dianna, my show is *Law and Order*." Thanks, Dick, for joining our board so many years ago, doing your own good work for conservation, and for that very nice gift, despite my TV ignorance!

Wanting to introduce my new friend, Martha, to Maine Coast Heritage Trust's long-time former board chair, I haul her across the lawn. Ed, who is also a prominent lawyer and former Yale athletic director, stands with my husband at the Maine Coast Heritage Trust summer celebration. Martha is attractive perfection in every manner. Ed smiles and exposes a toothless grin, as he is mid-point in dental work. We chat for a few minutes. As Martha and I drift back into the crowd, I hear Ed say to Ben, "Wow. Who the hell was that?" Fortunately, with her sense of humor and history of generosity, recognition was not essential for Martha Stewart.

IDEAS FOR VOLUNTEER ENGAGEMENT

On we go to some ideas for volunteer engagement, just in case you need some help. You can come up with many opportunities to volunteer. As you reach out to enrich your life through giving back to the world and her creatures, a perfect fit is out here waiting for you. A sample of opportunities is listed below.

American Farmland Trust:
"saves the land that sustains us by protecting farmland, promoting sound farming practices, and keeping farmers on the land."

American Society for the Prevention of Cruelty of Animals:
provides "an effective means for the prevention of cruelty to animals throughout the United States."

Conservation Law Foundation:
"forges solutions to New England's biggest environmental challenges—climate change, clean water, healthy communities—for all."

Cornell Lab of Ornithology:
"interprets and conserves the earth's biological diversity through research, education, and citizen science focused on birds." At the Lab, "scientists, conservationists, engineers, educators, and students all work together for a common purpose: to understand birds and other wildlife, to involve the public in scientific discovery, and to use our knowledge to protect our planet."

The Cornell Lab's magazine, *Living Bird,* and its partner, *Northern Woodlands,* suggest some things you can do quickly to assist birds: keep your birdfeeders clean to prevent disease; plant native plants; and keep your cats indoors. Great Backyard Bird Count (birdcount.org) helps researchers at National Audubon Society and Cornell Lab of

Ornithology through citizen scientist observations of birds, and Project Feeder Watch engages volunteers to count birds at their feeders over the winter. What an incentive this is to study and help the avian population, even when we are unable to get outdoors.

Environmental Defense Fund:
"preserve(s) the natural systems on which all life depends. Guided by science and economics, we find practical and lasting solutions to the most serious environmental problems."

Forest Society of Maine:
"conserves Maine's forestlands to sustain their ecological, economic, cultural, and recreational values."

Friends of Acadia:
"preserves, protects, and promotes stewardship of the outstanding natural beauty, ecological vitality, and distinctive cultural resources of Acadia National Park and surrounding communities for the inspiration and enjoyment of current and future generations." From grooming the winter trails network, to cleaning the roadsides of trash, to raking leaves from the carriage roads' ditches, to registering people for events—FOA has a job for you.

Friends of Virgin Islands National Park:
"advances the protection and preservation of the natural and cultural resources of Virgin Islands National Park and promotes the responsible enjoyment of this unique national treasure while educating and inspiring adults and children to be stewards of the environment." One important way to help this Friends group is to assist in the maintenance of the trail network, where tropic vegetation needs to regularly be cut back.

Greenpeace:
"is the leading independent campaigning organization that uses peaceful protest and creative communication to expose global environmental problems and promote solutions that are essential to a green and peaceful future."

Island Institute:
"works to sustain Maine's island and remote coastal communities, and exchanges ideas and experiences to further the sustainability of communities here and elsewhere."

Maine Coast Heritage Trust:
"conserves and stewards Maine's coastal lands and islands for their renowned scenic beauty, ecological value, outdoor recreational opportunities, and contribution to community well-being. MCHT provides statewide conservation leadership through its work with land trusts, coastal communities, and other partners." MCHT has protected 322 islands, conserved 150,000 acres of land, created 81 miles of trails, and maintains 129 preserves.

Maine Farmland Trust:
"is a member-powered statewide organization that protects farmland, supports farmers, and advances the future of farming."

Mount Desert Island Biological Laboratory:
"improves(s) human health and well-being through basic research, education, and development ventures that transform discoveries into cures."

National Audubon Society:
conserves and restores "natural ecosystems focusing on birds, other wildlife, and their habitats for the benefit of humanity and the earth's biological diversity." Volunteer opportunities at Audubon are numerous.

National Park Foundation:
NPF is the "official charitable partner of the National Park Service." They are connected with all of the national parks across the United States and can help you to develop a relationship with one near you.

National Parks Conservation Association:
protects and enhances "America's National Park System for present and future generations."

National Wildlife Federation:
inspires "Americans to protect wildlife for our children's future." Two of NWF's many compelling programs are Garden for Wildlife, which

connects gardeners to native plants beneficial to wildlife in their zip-code area and its native tree program, Trees for Wildlife. Your garden can become a NWF Certified Wildlife Habitat through providing habitat that nurtures wildlife (www.nwf.org/WildlifeGardenDesign).

New England Forestry Foundation:
"strives to serve and unite people and organizations across the region to support the long-term health of New England's forests, and to guarantee their continued environmental, recreational, and economic benefits for all New Englanders."

Northern Woodlands:
seeks to "advance a culture of forest stewardship in the Northeast and to increase understanding of and appreciation for the natural wonders, economic productivity, and ecological integrity of the region's forests."

Ocean Conservancy:
"educates and empowers citizens to take action on behalf of the ocean. From the Arctic to the Gulf of Mexico to the halls of Congress, Ocean Conservancy brings people together to find solutions for our water planet. Informed by science, our work guides policy and engages people in protecting the ocean and its wildlife for future generations."

Oceana:
"is dedicated to protecting and restoring our oceans on a global scale."

Open Space Institute:
is "a national conservation organization that works with towns and community organizations interested in creating community forests," according to its president, Jennifer Melville, in an interview with *Northern Woodlands*. Melville explains, "Key to the definition of a community forest is protection."[78]

Sailors for the Sea:
educates and engages "the boating community in the worldwide protection of the oceans."

Schoodic Institute at Acadia National Park:
Schoodic Institute "is committed to guiding present and future generations to greater understanding and respect for nature by providing

research and learning opportunities through its outstanding Acadia National Park setting, unique coastal Maine facilities, and innovative partnership programs."

As an example of a specific volunteer experience that can have national significance, we take a look at the Institute's Bird Ecology Laboratory. Seth Benz, Director of the Bird Ecology Laboratory at Schoodic Institute, points out the importance of Schoodic's eastern Maine location as a refueling stop for migrating birds, where researchers and citizen scientists study, band, and collect stool samples from about 60 species each year. The synergy of combining professional research efforts with those of citizen scientists is particularly evident at the Institute, where studies focus on the broad range of bird relationships in nature—their feeding ecology, their movements and migratory patterns, their navigation in the night sky, their interactions with other species, and how all this has changed over time and will change more in the future. Banding studies at Schoodic include songbirds like dark-eyed juncos, golden-crowned kinglets, red-breasted nuthatches, white-throated sparrows, hermit thrushes, black-throated warblers, blackpoll warblers, and common yellowthroats. SeaWatch volunteers track loons, gannets, mergansers, cormorants, and other seabirds. Benz points out that birds are the ecosystem's harbingers of change and that counting them is important, particularly given that birds have declined by 50% over 60 years.

An important partner of the Schoodic Institute Bird Ecology Laboratory is the Cornell Lab of Ornithology, one of the world's greatest ornithological institutions and a champion of citizen science. This partnership brings resources to the Bird Ecology Laboratory in the form of expertise and shared grants, and it facilitates dissemination of research done at Acadia. The Cornell Lab, at over 100 years old, has long recognized the "duality of birds as tools for research and scientific training on the one hand, and for communication and inspiration on the other," according to its director, Louis Fitzpatrick. If your interests focus on birds, Cornell and partners like Schoodic Institute have a volunteer spot for you.

Sierra Club:

The mission is "to explore, enjoy, and protect the planet; to practice and promote the responsible use of the earth's ecosystems and resources; to educate and enlist humanity to protect and restore the quality of the natural and human environment; and to use all lawful means to carry out those objectives."

The Conservation Fund:
The purpose of The Conservation Fund is "to balance the protection of America's natural resources with economic development. The Fund endeavors to protect important landscapes having significant natural, historic, or open space value."

Trust for Public Land:
TPL's mission is "to create parks and protect land for people, ensuring healthy, livable communities for generations to come."

U.S. Fish and Wildlife Service:
is an agency within the federal government's Department of the Interior whose mission is "working with others to conserve, protect, and enhance fish, wildlife, plants, and their habitats for the continuing benefit of the American people."

Vermont Center for Ecostudies:
"promotes wildlife conservation across the Americas using the combined strength of scientific research and citizen engagement."

World Wildlife Fund:
WWF's mission is "to stop the degradation of the planet's natural environment and to build a future in which people live in harmony with nature by: conserving the world's biological diversity, ensuring that the use of renewable natural resources is sustainable, and promoting the reduction of pollution and wasteful consumption."

Xerces Society:
"works to protect invertebrates and their habitats."

All of Your Area's Local Land Trusts:
Examples for my area include Blue Hill Heritage Trust, Downeast Coastal Conservancy, Downeast Lakes Land Trust, and Frenchman Bay Conservancy.

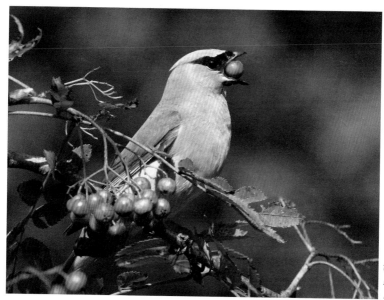

Leslie Clapp

Garden for Wildlife: Cedar Waxwing with Mountain Ash Fruit.

OTHER WAYS WE CAN HELP THE WORLD
AND HER CREATURES[52, 53, 54, 55, 57, 60, 71]

**What Can We Do to Help with Ecological Mismatch
and Climate Change Issues?**

1) Educate yourself or engage in a citizen science group where you can learn how native and invasive plant species disperse fruit and how birds, insects, and plant life cycles are changing.

2) Study the interaction of birds, insects, and plants.

3) Visit specific locations each day to observe and record the presence and abundance of flowers, fruits, birds, and insects.

4) Plant perennial and annual milkweeds to restore the food source of the monarch butterfly. Contact the Xerces Society[57] for further information.

5) Record information about and photograph birds and invertebrates eating flowers or fruits in those locations to provide evidence for study.

What Can We Do to Help to Eradicate Invasive Species?

1) Become familiar with the invasive plants of your region.
2) Object to the sale of invasive plants if you see them in nurseries. At home and in your community, replace invasive plants with noninvasive plants and shrubs that attract wildlife.
3) Do not allow invasive plants to flower and eradicate them by digging out or covering for an extended period, bagging and destroying any refuse.
4) Plant native species.
5) Volunteer for or organize community eradication efforts.
6) Assist in educating others. Inquire about local planting efforts; become engaged so that you can influence plantings.

What Can We Do to Assist the Pollinators?

1) Become familiar with the pollinators of your region and help to educate others regarding the threats to pollinators.
2) Plant gardens friendly to bees and other pollinators.
3) Provide pesticide-free water sources, use no pesticides, and remember that pesticides and pollinators do not mix.
4) Boycott stores that sell treated plants.
5) Pass on these words from the Xerces Society for Invertebrate Conservation's website about neonicotinoids (insecticides that can kill bees) and bear in mind the fact that:
"Neonicotinoids are found throughout the landscape in areas where they were not directly applied. Here are three ways neonicotinoids interact with the environment and can impact invertebrates:
Plant Uptake: Plants take up neonicotinoids, spreading the chemical through plant tissues, potentially exposing insects that contact pollen, nectar, or other plant tissue.
Dust from Coated Seed: Neonicotinoids are released in dust from coated seeds during mechanized planting. This dust can move off-site, exposing bees or contaminating non-target sites.
Persistence: Most neonicotinoids are long-lived, persisting for months to years after an application. Shrubs and trees may

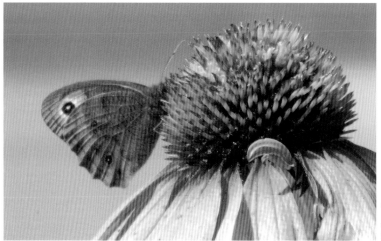

Melissa Savage

A Reciprocal Arrangement: Moth on Echinacea.

remain harmful, and residues in soil can be taken up by new plants."

6) Allow dandelions and clovers to grow in yards, keep meadows with wildflowers mowed every 1-2 years, and keep edges with brambles such as wild blackberry for bee nesting.

7) Avoid hybrid garden plants that do not provide pollen and nectar.

8) Encourage attention to climate change issues.

As we move through life, the piece of it that we give to others represents an opportunity to provide meaning and satisfaction as it takes us outside ourselves and puts us to work on behalf of the common good. Chances are that you are already giving much of yourself to other people and causes. When I consider my circle of friends and what they are doing for the world, I am in awe. Thank you all for your generous-spirited work on behalf of the natural world and her creatures.

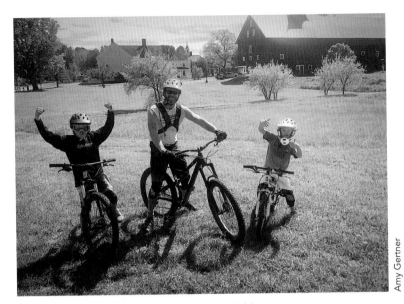

Join and Inspire the Children.

Amy Gertner

11

MODELING FOR THE NEXT GENERATION

"Nature holds the key to our aesthetic, intellectual,
cognitive, and even spiritual satisfaction."
E.O. Wilson

Modeling for the next generation means setting an example that will encourage them to lead healthy and satisfying lives, finding their route to making the transformational power of the natural world last a lifetime, and helping the world along the way. To do this, we need to start early. Like anything else, whether the task is learning to ski or speak a foreign language, the young ones are more likely to follow our example related to engaging with the green outdoors if we expose them from a young age and on a regular basis to all of the elements we have looked at in this book. It can be a natural thing to go outside instead of plunk down in front of a machine; to nurture the world and her creatures, rather than acting "me first no matter who or what it hurts;" to choose vegetables and fruits instead of candy as treats, if you understand where your food comes from and that you can grow some yourself; to walk instead of ride or to run instead of walk; to take the time for quiet contemplation and relaxation, instead of jamming in as much as one can as fast as possible; to reach out to form meaningful relationships with others, instead of turning our backs; and to give back in appreciation for what we have been given through volunteerism, rather than feeling entitled.

A cherished interaction in a quiet eastern Maine cove presents a perfect example of giving back. We watch a lobster boat approaching, clearly planning to come alongside our boat. Lobsters sound like a treat, and Ben goes below for his wallet. Two children and their parents grab lobsters and hold them out to us, as the dad explains that these lobsters were caught by his kids, who have worked in the trade for the summer. We say we are delighted to buy some. "Oh, no," he says, "this is lobsterman's trick-or-treat and the kids are treating you. Pay it forward." The kids look a little disappointed, but they put on a good show, as we thank them enthusiastically. What a shining lesson these parents taught their children. We send a contribution to their school library, with credit to the "lobster kids" for their generosity. Later, we receive a huge card with messages from all of the children in the school. In the corner, I see two names with a note, "We are the lobster ones."

This generation of children is faced with challenges much different than the ones that we grew up with. According to the *National Survey on Drug Use and Health*, conducted by the U.S. Department of Health and Human Services in 2006, 7.9% of adolescents aged 12 to 17 reported at least one depressive episode.[79] Diagnostic criteria of the Diagnostic and Statistical Manual of Mental Disorders-IV (DSM-IV) defines a major depressive episode as "a period of two weeks or longer during which there is either a depressed mood or loss of interest or pleasure, and at least four other symptoms that reflect a change in functioning, like problems with sleep, eating, energy, concentration, or self image."[80] By 2015, according to the National Institute of Health, 12.5% of children reported at least one depressive episode within the last year.[81] That is 3 million children. Of similar concern are reports that by 2015, 25% of adolescents in the age group from 13 to 18, or 6.3 million children, had experienced an anxiety disorder,[81] with too many of those releasing their pain through self-harm. How can we give this generation a hand?

Helping troubled children and all children to channel their energy into positive engagements exactly like those we have been reviewing can be of great help. Like their older counterparts, they respond to positive interaction and activities with their family and friends. If they are struggling, the whole family needs to work together, as sometimes the home environment can be tweaked to be healthier for all. Evaluating how changes in diet and exercise habits could have positive impact is an important part of that. Encouragement to join us in engaging deeply with the natural world and her creatures should be an invitation we offer often and start early.

Every child, and every adult who harbors an inner child, should have experiences with the natural world and her creatures. How can we help to provide such opportunities to those within our reach while also enriching the world and ourselves? Walking along a Maine seashore

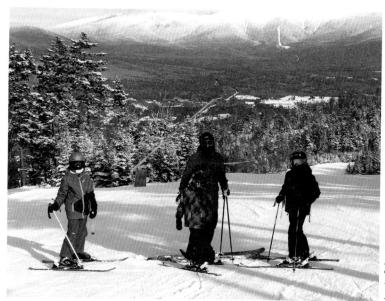

Outside Early at Bretton Woods.

with a troupe of children, I gently lift the rockweed to uncover the hidden world beneath. Startled by our shadows, delicate baby crabs slip into the adjacent tide pool to retreat under rock crevices, soon creeping out to feed once more. Anthropods, what I once thought of as tiny shrimp, wriggle in the rockweed and swim in large numbers in the tide pool. We put our faces down close to the weed and pool, rest our faces on the warm granite, close our eyes, and listen. It is so quiet. In the stillness, there is the sound of the sea lapping against the shore and stones tinkling as each wave retreats. A raspy-throated raven calls, and the distinctive cry of an osprey reminds us of the nest we spotted earlier. We breathe in deeply of the scent of the sea and the salty rockweed, open our eyes and again look down into the tide pool. Barnacles open and close, feeding with their little tentacles, as we notice a small anemone seeming to wave at us.

From the tide pool, we walk over the ledges and amongst the rockweed, picking up bottles, cans, and other refuse. It is appalling to see

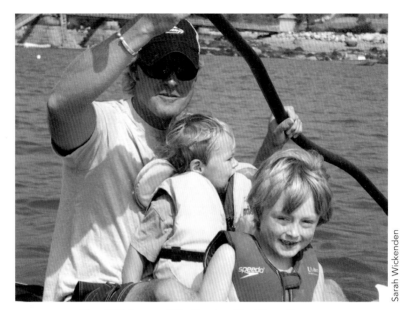

Sarah Wickenden

They Will Become Who You Are: Start Them Young.

how much trash can be found on the seaside. This provides the opportunity to talk with the children about their own ability to impact what litters our planet and how even a walk on the shore offers a chance to do something important for our vulnerable world. I tell the story of what one sees out on the open ocean. Swimming amidst a sea of trash are giant turtles, multi-hued dolphin fish, whales, and many other creatures that can mistake the bags, balloons, and yogurt containers for edibles. We talk about how we should use our plastics and how we can recycle more effectively, helping to protect the sea creatures. "Every little bit helps," one boy shouts out.

Finding opportunities for even young children to learn how to be less introspective or self-centered, to instead volunteer and give back in thanks for what they have been given, promises them great rewards. Our children watch us carefully. Let's be sure that what they see is what we want them to become.

CONCLUSION

The loggers balance on downed tree trunks, half sunk in ponds and marshes, soaking up the warming rays in preparation for feeding. These loggers do not fell trees or fuel themselves on hearty sandwiches. They are the painted turtles, harbingers of the short Northeast spring and summer.

One promising April day, ten loggers, from quarter-sized to bowl-sized, line a log near Acadia's Witch Hole Pond. Through the trunks of white pine and spruce, I peek through and try to get a little closer, wishing I had my camera. The slap of a beaver's tail startles the turtles, and all but one shoot into the water. That one little turtle hangs onto his log as it sways in the waves, riding it out while the others gradually begin poking their heads up through the water. We are a bit like that. Some of us panic and come undone when the going gets tough, while others persevere through daunting times. We marvel at those who hang on after encountering the most difficult of circumstances.

How do we get from that state of worry to a place where we can gather up our coping mechanisms and bolster our resilience? Or, how can we plan for a future when our bodies and our minds are not quite what they are right now? A measured approach might not solve our problems or turn back our biological clocks, but it can take us a long way toward feeling that we have more control over our lives.

Let's begin by focusing on the Five V's again, beginning with **Visualization**, and recalling a relaxing place from our memory or imagination. Write or record a detailed description of that place and the creatures that you find there. I have done that here.

We are standing on the bank of an evergreen-ringed pond that is filled with white water lilies. A warm breeze slightly ruffles the water as a bullfrog gives a low croak and a thrush calls from the woods. Examining the lilies across the pond, we discover that one patch is not white, but pink. There are five pink ones amidst many hundreds of whites, calling out their individual differences. How fortunate we feel to be in this place, in this time, as we look below the water's surface, where the lilies' roots reach deep into the mud. A minnow glides by. Is it a trout? We will find out later by checking online. Moving along the bank, we watch a group of whirligig beetles skittering around the water's surface as two damselflies hover above. Out on the pond a frog suns himself, perched on a lily pad while his mate shows only her bulbous eyes and green snout above the water's surface. We contemplate what it must be like to be a frog, swimming under the lily pads past tadpoles, minnows, and the occasional turtle, then sticking one's head up to greet the sunshine.

Now read your passage aloud and mine as well, if you choose. How do you feel?

Let's go outside or close to a living thing indoors, right now. I am walking out to look at a bold pink rocket snapdragon. What are you looking at? Let's look at the details. I see rows of blossoms down the snapdragon stalk, each one a little reservoir of pollen. Here comes a bumblebee. I watch him do something I have never seen before. He climbs inside the snapdragon blossom, disappears completely as it snaps shut, and then backs out, furry bottom first. Now I see more bumblebees doing the same thing. How could I have lived nearly seven decades, explored so much of nature, and never noticed this fascinating behavior? Guess I just didn't take the time. What are you seeing now in your bit of the natural world? Are there some things you could still explore and learn about if you give yourself the gift of time? Can you build some of these into visualizations for future use?

Sometimes being slowed down by age, illness, or overwhelming responsibilities can have a silver lining. Recovery from surgeries over the years has given me the time to concentrate on the details of life and make them part of my daily routine. Every second of every day is a blessing that I think about and express thanks for each morning. If you focus on detail and make it a part of your life, giving thanks and visualizing that for which you are thankful, it is a powerful engagement. Let's try it, adding other things for which you are thankful whenever you want. Each time you read a bold-type word, close your eyes, and see what is in your mind's eye or think about how you are feeling. I let my mind drift to one of a particular set of creatures or other things. For instance, for "butterflies" right now I see a monarch butterfly and for "moth" I see a luna moth. Or, if I am thinking of birds, an image of a different bird drifts into my mind's eye, depending upon whether I am focusing on sky, earth and soil, or waters. Here is my thank-you script.

*Thank you for the **sky**, the **universe**, the **planets**, the **sun**, the **moon**, the **stars**, the **Earth**, the **clouds**, and thank you for the **air that we breathe**. Thank you for the **sunshine**, the **rain**, the **snow**, the **sleet**, the **hail**, and the **breezes**.*

*Thank you for the **creatures of the sky**—the **birds**, the **bees**, the **butterflies**, the **moths**, the **bats**, the **insects**, and all the other creatures of the sky. I will do the best that I can to help to care for your world and your creatures.*

*Thank you for the **Earth** and for the **soil**. Thank you for the **geological features**. Thank you for the things you grow on the Earth and in the soil. Thank you for the **fruits**, the **berries**, the **vegetables**, the **trees** and the **shrubs**, the **flowers** and the **weeds**, the **lichens** and the **mosses**, and all the other things that grow on your Earth and in your soil. I will do the best that I can to help to care for your world and your creatures.*

*Thank you for the **creatures of the Earth and of the soil**. Thank you for the **reptiles**, the **amphibians**, the **mammals**, the **birds**, the **worms**, the **insects**, and all the other creatures of your Earth and of your soil. I will do the best that I can to help to care for your world and your creatures.*

*Thank you for the **waters, fresh and salt**. Thank you for the **lakes** and the **ponds**, the **rivers** and the **streams**, the **bogs** and the **brooks**, the **marshes** and the **swamps**, the **estuaries** and the **salt ponds**, and thank you for the **oceans** wide that bind us all together.*

*Thank you for the **creatures of your waters, fresh and salt**. Thank you for the **fishes**, the **birds**, the **mammals**, the **reptiles**, the **amphibians**, the **worms**, the **crustaceans**, the **insects**, and all the other creatures of your waters, fresh and salt. I will do the best that I can to help to care for your world and your creatures.*

Thank you for my family and for my friends. Thank you for strength-
ening them and caring for them physically, emotionally, and spiritually,
helping them to do the best that they can to help to care for your world and
your creatures. I will do the best that I can to help to care for each of them.

Now write down all of the words in bold type, and next to them
write the first image that comes into mind for each word. Then, practice visualizing each image in as much detail as possible. Sometimes
you might be interested to find yourself getting an image of a creature,
place, plant, or person from another time in your life. When I closed
my eyes a few minutes ago, an image came to me of my little black
Booby Rabbit—a pet named when I was nine years old and did not
know why everyone laughed at his name. Booby came to me in great
detail in my mind's eye. I could feel him sitting in my child's lap as I
stroked his ears, and I could vividly recall the scent of the grain that
he ate. I remember how important that bunny was at a time when I
did not feel safe in the world, each day questioning my mortality. He
helped to keep me in the present. As you move through the bold-typed
words, perhaps interesting images and feelings will come to you as well.

Let's turn now to the subject of **Venturing Forth**—adventures in
the green world where we can build memories and visual images to
which we can return in our mind's eye whenever we choose. I will share
some of the details of a recent adventure along the Maine Coast and a
bit of what you might choose to explore by car or on the water as well.
As I describe this expedition, I will also bring in the **Volunteerism** piece
of the Five V's, as the places I went were preserved and are stewarded in
large part thanks to volunteers.

The journey begins on the Witch Hole Pond and Paradise Hill
loop in Acadia National Park, a carriage road that I have run, hiked,
skied, and biked hundreds of times. Thanks to volunteers from Friends
of Acadia and others, this carriage road and the rest of the network are

kept clear of debris. In winter, volunteers groom the roads for cross-country skiing, due to an endowment created by Leila Bright, who hiked and skied Acadia throughout her long life. Others have contributed their time, energy, and dollars to ensure further maintenance. The journey connects us to many types of properties that you can access: federal lands, private places that owners are willing to share, land trust properties, community spaces, and your own backyard.

The Witch Hole/Paradise Hill loop is one of the most magnificent short trails in the park system, as it provides several pond and marsh sightings, an abundance of forests, and distant ocean vistas of islands and the Schoodic District of Acadia. On this run, I am hopeful that I will see some wildlife. At each pond and marsh, I will pause to take a closer look. The first sunshine-drenched pond provides a glimpse of painted turtles on their log—larger now than those I saw last spring. My foot squishes in the mud and startles a leopard frog that leaps into the pond, strokes its way to the bottom, and sticks its head into the muck. Its back legs and bottom are in full view causing me to wonder, if I were a hungry raccoon, just how long that frog would last. Little minnows dart about, and an interesting iridescent bluish-black wasp with long brown antennae captures my attention. He is a great black wasp, feeding himself while pollinating and removing plant pests that he will feed to his young.

I run some more and notice movement in the next pond. Expecting a beaver, as numerous lodges dot the ponds of Acadia National Park, I am astounded to watch four large otters sliding up onto a muddy outcropping; bounding back into the water to splash, dive, and play; and then clamoring onto the bank again. For quite some time I watch, stopping other runners, hikers, and bikers who join me in this exciting observation. I offer to take a family photo for a group of bikers, and then off I go to complete my run. Racing along, I reflect on the gathering of Maine Conservation Voters at Allison and Steve Sullens' house a few days ago. Generous in many ways, this young family has opened their home and their hearts to encourage others to support conservation interests. Keynote addresses are presented by Lucas St. Clair and Michael Boland, the owner of several Bar Harbor area restaurants where he and his wife, Dee Swords, regularly host events for area non-profits, *pro bono*. Lucas is the son of philanthropist, environmentalist, and Burt's Bees founder, Roxanne Quimby, who has donated 89,000 acres for the Katahdin Woods and Waters National Monument and made many other important gestures on behalf of conservation. In his own right, Lucas is a great conservation leader—an inspirational man who with his wife, Yemaya, is dedicated to the protection of the natural world. Yemaya speaks of her own early enchantment with nature as she examined aquatic life in the shallows. In the crowd are dozens of others who give generously in so many ways. Anne Green has taken on the chairmanship of Friends of Acadia; Cody VanHeerden and Cynthia Livingston sit on the board of Schoodic Institute at Acadia National Park; Lili Pew is on the board of College of the Atlantic and is a former chair of FOA; Lillie Johnson works tirelessly on behalf of conservation in many ways, including as a Council member of Maine Coast Heritage Trust; Caroline Pryor works on behalf of conservation and wounded wildlife; Hank Schmelzer is former President of the Maine Community Foundation and a volunteer in many capacities; Steve Sullens is an instrumental board member at Maine Coast Heritage Trust; Clara Baker works on behalf of Island Housing Trust; Linda Paine shares her extraordinary knowledge of plants in many directions; Lucas St. Clair is president of the board of Elliotsville Plantation…the list goes on and on—volunteers, each doing the best that they can to help the world—digging out the ditches in the park, hauling tables as they help with events, brainstorming, making phone calls, cooking meals for the needy, balancing budgets, assisting Hospice patients, and endeavoring in so many ways to try to make a difference. By the end of my run, I am in awe of the many people who have given so much. Our country is full of these generous-spirited souls. Chances are, you are one of them.

From the Mount Desert District of Acadia, we travel to the Park's Schoodic District where more marvels of the natural world abound, as do more examples of volunteerism. Hiking along the new Schoodic

Woods trails, we are so grateful to the thoughtful visionary donors who protected this land that abutted Acadia National Park and then gave it to the Park, complete with new trails, a campground, and a visitor's center. As we hike along, discussing this amazing gift, a flutter in the brush attracts our attention. A spruce grouse is fanning his speckled tail in full territorial glory. The grouse continues to forage, much like a chicken, as we walk along a few feet away. Later in the day, we tell the spruce grouse story to Vicki and Alan Goldstein, first-rate volunteers for hospitals, animal shelters, the Farnsworth Museum, and Schoodic Institute, where Alan is the chairman of the board. We all reflect on one of the most remarkable volunteers around, Campbell "Buzz" Scott, who dedicates his life and his salary to OceansWide, a nonprofit he created to bring kids from New York's Village Community School, Maine's Sumner High School, and other schools to camps at Schoodic Institute, where they learn scuba science, observe bird ecology, work with remotely operated underwater vehicles (ROVs), and help to clean the ocean floor of ghost lobster traps. One day we hope Buzz will have the new Falcon ROV and the research vessel that are his dream.

As we move along the coast, a different kind of adventure in the natural world is offered at Petit Manan National Wildlife Refuge, where boardwalk bridges of recycled CorrectDeck route hikers past informative naturalist signs. There we spot a lengthy garter snake, a ruffed grouse, Bonaparte gulls, eagles, and two thrushes. One sign quotes the namesake of the Hollingsworth Trail, John Hollingsworth, who advised students of nature to "simplify, simplify, simplify." Hollingsworth is memorialized for photographing over 400 national wildlife refuges. Reflecting on this fact, we remind ourselves of how important it is to go deep into the details of the natural world. Heading east from Petit Manan on the ocean, we are treated to sightings of puffins and razorbill auks. Later, meandering through the islands, we talk about Ben's efforts on behalf of The Conservation Fund as it worked to preserve eastern Maine's Bold Coast, where steep cliffs plummet ninety feet down to the sea. Pride overcomes me as I think about the many remarkable things he and others have done to preserve this coastline and its islands.

After exploring two different kinds of federal lands, we row to one of many undeveloped islands in private ownership. We appreciate the opportunity to sit on a lovely sand spit overlooking Narraguagus Bay, where large flocks of herring gulls follow lobster boats, planning to capture some of the discarded bait fish.

The next destination is very different, as it is protected through a conservation easement to Maine Coast Heritage Trust. Although we do not go ashore, we paddle board and row along the pristine shoreline, grateful that the owner chose to conserve this special place. Nearby Flint Island and Shipstern Island were protected by The Nature Conservancy prior to the formation of Maine Coast Heritage Trust. We recall that Little Nash Island is a place where sheep once roamed around the lighthouse. Ben and I owned "island sheep," remnants of flocks placed on Maine islands to keep vegetation low. How those sheep made it through winters with no human help is a lingering question, but many of us did adopt the island sheep when they were finally removed in the 1970s. The wild creatures that were their companions were surely better-suited for island life.

Following exploration by paddle boards of Bunker Cove, our favorite spot in the Roque Island archipelago, we learn of a forecast for eight-foot swells and high winds—remnants of Hurricane Harvey's devastating visit to the Houston area. Taking a preventative approach to our long sail home, in the same manner that we take a preventative approach to health care, we err on the side of caution and head for a safe harbor several hours away. Stave Island is out of the swell and gives us the opportunity to hike on the shoreline of this magnificent island, where several parcels have been protected and are now owned by Maine Coast Heritage Trust as a preserve. The public access allowed by an MCHT Preserve grants hikers, kayakers, picnickers, and boaters the enjoyment of an island visit. Your local land trusts are likely to offer similar opportunities for exploration of preserved lands, although all conserved properties do not allow public access. Regarding those, viewing the undeveloped and protected green spaces from a distance is value enough.

This tale of venturing forth and volunteerism might lead you to explore your immediate environment or the federal, state, and community resources that are within your reach. Perhaps you will also recall past adventures in the natural world that are etched within your mind and are ready to be incorporated into visualizations.

From Stave Island, we head for home, where my early fall garden greets me. This and the space inside our home is my immediate environment—the **Venturing Forth** to which I turn when I cannot go farther afield. It is a nurturing place to which I can turn to use each of the **Five V's** we have focused on in this book. Here I engage in **Vetting** the healthy approaches that fit my life at a given time. Sometimes I make the wrong choices—exercising before the stitches are healed, eating the ice cream when my pants are too tight, not calling a friend whom I have not seen for too long—but, I will keep on trying. I can still move forward to a healthier place. Here I can continue to **Volunteer**, even if all I can do is talk on the phone. Here I can **Visualize** all of those remarkable places and creatures from my memory and my imagination that can help me to feel that my connection to nature goes on and on. And, from this place, I can participate in the **Viewing** of others' successes, learning as I go, despite aging's effects or other life challenges.

These things are so important—**Volunteering, Visualizing, Vetting, Venturing Forth**, and **Viewing**—even if they all happen in a microcosm. You can take whatever immediate environment you have and make it a nurturing and welcoming space that can bring you joy and access to nature and her creatures during the periods when you are not able to go farther afield.

My immediate environment is a nurturing one—a place where I can **Venture Forth, Visualize, Vet Healthy Choices,** and **Volunteer.** I can also **View Others' Successes** as they find ways to continue to connect with the natural world and her creatures, even when life challenges and aging issues interfere. This question was posed to several people, "When you have faced medical issues, stressors, or the aging process, how have you continued to maintain a connection to the natural world and her creatures?" This response is a representative sample:

Former Superintendent of Acadia National Park, Sheridan Steele: "When I cannot sleep or when I am facing a particularly stressful situation, I concentrate on some of my wonderful experiences—usually from times spent in national parks like Rocky Mountain, Acadia, Arches, Zion, Yosemite, and Black Canyon. I am especially fond of experiences of contemplation on the shore of a spectacular high mountain lake like Sky Pond, or walking along a beautiful clear mountain stream like Calypso Cascades and Ouzel Falls in Rocky Mountain National Park, or hiking by moonlight across slick-rock desert to Delicate Arch in Arches National Park, or holding onto thick chains as we climbed Angel's Landing in Zion. Returning to these beautiful places (in my mind) brings instant relaxation and a sense of serenity and peace."

It seems fitting, as I write the final pages of this book, that the early dawn hours find me paddle boarding among the protected islands of Maine's Eggemoggin Reach. A hint of fall is in the air, and I need an extra layer today. As I skim across the smooth surface of the Reach, a porpoise approaches to dive beneath my board and continue the search for mackerel. This time he doesn't linger, going about his business of surfacing and feeding. Harbor seals are around, too, poking their heads up and following me occasionally. A lone eagle soars high above the Torrey

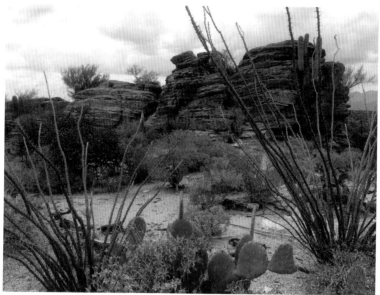

Dianna Emory

New Adventures: Saguaro National Park.

Island shore, as three young osprey fly not so far away. This time, they are safe. All seems to be in harmony with the wild things of the Reach today. I wish the world were in the same place, and I pray for peace and sanity, as my resounding prayer for those suffering the effects of recent hurricanes, discrimination, or other pains also echoes in my mind.

The sun is rising, filtering through light clouds as I speak my thank-you prayer for all that is around me in the natural world; for the opportunity to be here—so much longer than I ever expected; and for the ability to do the best that I can to help to care for God's world and her creatures. Shafts of sunlight pierce the clouds, casting a golden glow across the water, as I express thanks for the spiritual, physical, and emotional strengthening of friends and family members. I pray for this world to have many more sunrises.

AUTHOR'S NOTE

An unusual experience related to impending crisis rose out of my sleep and served as the catalyst to complete this book.

My husband, Ben, and I lie sleeping in a remote anchorage, on the island-studded coast of Maine. I wake suddenly to full alertness brought on by the intense pain that has troubled my stomach day after day for months. After a lifetime of eluding the cancer that first struck me as an infant, I am prepared for the worst. No medical advice has been sought—quite unlike me—as I am so convinced that this is bad. Soaked in sweat and doubled up in pain, I promise that I will do my best, regardless of the hand that is dealt. Ben snores quietly beside me, unaware of my unshared fears. I feel a deep sadness at the thought that my time has likely come and that I will need to leave cherished family and friends behind. Some solace comes from the promise of seeing those who earlier left this life. Then, out of the darkness, a palpable presence begins to fill our boat's aft cabin. Like a soft and feathery nest, I feel it all around me, soothing my senses, easing away tension, sinking deep into every fiber of my being. A strong message penetrates all. "Your time has not yet come. You have much to do here. Give back for what you are given." I drift off to the gentle lapping of the waves against the boat's hull, feeling peaceful and in love with the world. In the morning, I am refreshed and pain-free for the first time in many months. The pain does not return—not that day nor any day after. In thanks, I make a pledge to do all that I can to provide hope and inspiration to others, while acting on behalf of the natural world, through sharing the things that I know intimately.

That is the essence of this book.

ACKNOWLEDGMENTS

Thanks are extended to my conservation mentor and husband, Ben Emory, and to the many other conservation advocates who have impacted my life and the natural world through their example and generosity. They include Jay Espy, Tim Glidden, Dr. Mike Soukup, Dr. Paul Mayewski, Ken Olson, Sheridan Steele, Joe Kessler, Edith Dixon, Lillie Johnson, Phoebe Milliken, Ruth and Tris Colket, David and Susan Rockefeller, Roxanne Quimby, Dr. Steve Katona, Alan Goldstein, and so many others. Those who left this world too early, but whose impact is still felt, include Minerva Converse Kendall Warner, Ken Warner, Richard Rockefeller, Alan Hutchinson, Beth and Don Straus, Patricia and David Scull, Claire Shepley, and Norman Kilby. For their creative inspiration, affection, and generosity of spirit, many thanks to Melissa and Bethany Savage, and for his athletic inspiration and companionship, Thor Emory.

A special note of appreciation for their beautiful photographs is extended to Downeast Audubon President Leslie Clapp, retired Acadia National Park Superintendent Sheridan Steele, Sherry Streeter, David Manski, Bethany Savage, Melissa Savage, and Ben Emory.

For their encouragement and generous endorsements, many thanks to Roxana Robinson, Senator George Mitchell, Dr. Michael Soukup, Jill Soule, Dr. Robert Gossart, Lester and Joyce Coleman, Dr. Dan Poteet, Roy and Emily Van Vleck, Michelle Paisley, and Ellen Kappes. Queene Foster, my editor, Jane Crosen, my copyeditor, Claire MacMaster, my designer, and Spencer Smith of Seapoint Books, my publisher, are appreciated for their assistance with this project.

Many thanks to my mother, Ruth Warner Kilby Gruninger, who has been there through it all and to my sister, Lois Kilby-Chesley, who joined me early in life.

The biggest thanks of all goes to God for bringing so many wonderful friends and family members into my life and for giving me access to all that nature holds. The challenges have been many, but they have guided me to treasure every moment and to better understand the plight of others and the natural world.

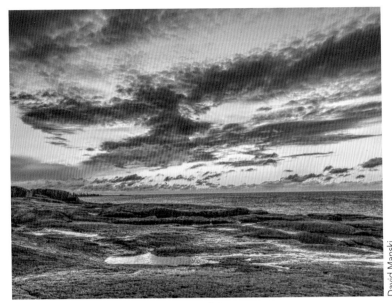

David Manski

A Promise of Hope.

This book is dedicated to our grandsons, Wyeth Schapiro, Finn Emory, Zander Schapiro, Carver Emory, and Porter Schapiro, and to the natural world that I hope they will steward.

DEFINITIONS

Cognitive Behavioral Therapy, as defined by Psych Central, is a "short-term, goal-oriented psychotherapy treatment that takes a hands-on, practical approach to problem-solving. Its goal is to change patterns of thinking or behavior that are behind people's difficulties, and so change the way they feel."

Creative Visualization, as defined by Wikipedia, is "the cognitive process of purposefully generating visual mental imagery, with eyes open or closed, simulating or recreating visual perception, in order to maintain, inspect, and transform those images, consequently modifying their associated emotions or feelings, with intent to experience a subsequent beneficial physiological, psychological, or social effect, such as expediting the healing of wounds to the body, minimizing physical pain, alleviating psychological pain including anxiety, sadness, and low mood, improving self-esteem or self-confidence, and enhancing the capacity to cope when interacting with others."

Green Environments, as defined by Kaplan in 1995, are "any environment that affords an individual the opportunity to view a more green type of scenery."

Green Exercise, as defined by Wikipedia, is "physical exercise undertaken in natural environments."

Guided Imagery, as defined by the U.S. Department of Health and Human Services, National Institutes of Health, is "a mind-body intervention by which a trained practitioner or teacher helps a participant or patient to evoke and generate mental images that simulate or re-create the sensory perception of sights, sounds, tastes, smells, movements, and images."

Holistic Health, as defined by the American Holistic Health Association, is "an approach to life. Rather than focusing on illness or specific parts of the body, this ancient approach to health considers the whole person and how he or she interacts with his or her environment. It emphasizes the connection of mind, body, and spirit."

Mind-Body Interventions, as defined by the National Center for Complementary and Integrative Health (a component of the National Institutes of Health) "employ a variety of techniques designed to facilitate the mind's capacity to affect bodily function and symptoms. They include guided imagery, guided meditation and forms of meditative praxis, hypnosis and hypnotherapy, and prayer, as well as art therapy, music therapy, and dance therapy." They "focus on the interaction between the brain, body, and behavior and are practiced with intention to use the mind to alter physical function and promote overall health and well-being."

Psychoneuroimmunology, as defined by Dr. Robert Ader who coined the term, is "the study of interactions between psychological, neurological, and immune systems."

REFERENCES

1   *The Wall Street Journal*, "Secrets of Successful Aging," June 20, 2005.

2   Cohen, Sheldon. *The Perceived Stress Scale*, 1983.

3   Mayo Clinic. *Patient Care and Health Information*. "Cognitive Behavioral Therapy," March 2, 2017 website, first posted February 23, 2016.

4   American Medical Association, American Psychological Association, American Society of Clinical Hypnosis, American Association for the Advancement of Science, World Federation of Mental Health.

5   Friedman, Thomas. *Thank You for Being Late*. 2016, 450.

6   *Subaru Drive*. Spring 2017, 20.

7   Seligman, Martin, and Deiner, Ed. "Beyond Money: Toward an Economy of Well Being," *Science in the Public Interest*, volume 5, number 1, University of Illinois.

8   Deiner, Ed, Emmons, Robert A., Larsen, Randy J., and Griffin, Sharon. Satisfaction with Life Scale. *Journal of Personality Assessment*, 57, 149-161.

9   Moskowitz, Judith. Research cited: "Personal Health: Positive Thinking May Improve Health," *Medinary*, posted March 27, 2017.

10 National Institutes of Health. *Clinical Trials*, posted May 22, 2016.

11 Moskowitz, Judith. "Positive Thinking May Improve Health," *Medinary*, posted on website March 27, 2017.

12 Levy, Becca. *Journal of Gerontology*. In Brody, Jane. " A Positive Outlook May Be Good for Your Health," *The New York Times*, March 28, 2017.

13 *The New York Times*. "Science Times," March 29, 2016.

14 Kuo, Frances E., and Taylor, Faber. "A Potential Natural Treatment for Attention-Deficit/Hyperactivity Disorder: Evidence from a National Study." *American Journal of Public Health, 94.9*, September 2004.

15 Puett, Robin. "How Does Exercising Outdoors vs. Indoors Influence Mental and Physical Wellbeing?" University of Maryland School of Public Health. Posted November 2014.

16 *The Wall Street Journal*. "Health Journal," May 10, 2005.

17 *Neuroscience and Biobehavioral Reviews*. February 2016.

18 *The New York Times*. "How Exercise Might Keep Depression at Bay," November 16, 2016.

19 *Journal of Psychiatric Review*. June 2016.

20 Kaplan, Rachael and Stephen. *The Experience of Nature: A Psychological Perspective*, Cambridge University Press, 1989.

21 Kelly, M. "Creature Comfort." *Health Sciences*, Spring 1988, 2-25.
22 Fouchaux, J. In J.S. Bland, *Animal-Facilitated Therapy: The Benefits of Equestrian Therapy for the Physically Handicapped with Cerebral Palsy*. University of North Colorado, 1982, 12.
23 Friedman and Katcher. In Arkow, P. "Pet Therapy: A Study of the Use of Companion Animals in Selected Therapies," The Humane Society of the Pikes Peak Region, 1982.
24 Levinson, B.M. *Pet-Oriented Child Psychotherapy*. Springfield, IL: Charles C. Thomas, 1972.
25 Katcher, A.H. "Interactions between People and Their Pets: Form and Function." In B. Fogle (Ed.), *Interrelations between People and Pets*. Springfield, IL: Charles C. Thomas, 1981, 41-67.
26 Beck, A.M., and Katcher, A.H., *Between Pets and People: The Importance of Animal Companionship*. New York: G.P. Putnam and Sons, 1983.
27 Riddick, C.C. " Health, Aquariums, and the Non-Institutionalized Elderly," *Marriage and Family Review, 8.*, 1985, 163-173.
28 Damon, J., and May, R. "The Effects of Pet Facilitated Therapy on Patients and Staff in an Adult Day Care Center," *Activities and Aging, 8*, 1986, 117-131.
29 McCullough, "The Pet as Prosthesis." In B. Fogle (Ed.), *Interrelations Between People and Pets,* 1981b, 101-103.
30 Mugford, R.A., and M'Comisky, J.G. "Some Recent Work on the Psychotherapeutic Value of Cage Birds with Old People." In R.S. Anderson (Ed.), *Pet Animals and Society,* 1975, 54-65.
31 Corson, S.A., Corson, E.O., and Gwynne, P.H. "Pet Facilitated Psychotherapy." In R.S. Anderson (Ed.), *Pet Animals and Society*, London: Bailliere Tindall, 1975, 19-36.
32 Kroodsma, Don. *Backyard Birdsong*, Cornell Lab Publishing Group, 2016.
33 Katcher, A.H., and Beck, A.M. (Eds.). *New Perspectives on Our Lives with Companion Animals*. Philadelphia: University of Pennsylvania Press, 1983, 412.
34 Jared, Peter. "Reap the Benefits of Gardening," *Martha Stewart Living*, March 2007.
35 Sorin, Fran. *Digging Deep: Unearthing Your Creative Roots through Gardening*, 2009.
36 Blair, Steven. *Active Living Every Day*, Human Kinetics Publishers, 2001.
37 Walls, Margaret. "Parks and Recreation in the United States, Local Park Systems," *Backgrounder*, June 2009.
38 Walls, Margaret. "Parks and Recreation in the United States, State Park

Systems," *Backgrounder*, January 2009.

39 National Parks Conservation Association Press Release, January 27, 2016.

40 National Parks Conservation Association Press Release, March 10, 2017.

41 National Parks Conservation Association Press Release, January 27, 2016.

42 Brody, Jane. "The Worst that Could Happen? Going Blind, People Say," *The New York Times*, February 21, 2017.

43 St. Germain, Tom. *A Walk in the Park*, Parkman Publications, 1993.

44 Kong, Dolores, and Ring, Dan. *Hiking Acadia National Park*. Falcon Guide, 2001, 2012.

45 Kong, Dolores, and Ring, Dan. *Best Easy Day Hikes, Acadia National Park*. Falcon Guide, 2011, 2017.

46 Fuentes, Jose. *National Wildlife*, April-May, 2010. From *Atmospheric Environment*.

47 Acadia National Park. From Green, et al., 2005.

48 Acadia National Park. From Chandler, et al., 2012.

49 Acadia National Park. From Miller-Rushing et al., 2008.

50 Acadia National Park. From Cahill et al., 2013.

51 Benz, Seth. Schoodic Institute presentation.

52 Mittelhauser, Glen H., Gregory, Linda L., Rooney, Sally C., and Weber, Jill E. *The Plants of Acadia National Park*, University of Maine Press, 2010, 5.

53 Yeoman, Barry. *National Wildlife*. "Going Native," April-May 2017, 31.

54 Tallamy, Doug. Lecture. From *Bringing Nature Home*, Timber Press, 2009.

55 Acadia National Park website. "Bees on the Brink," 2010.

56 The Natural History Center website. "Checklist of the Birds of Mount Desert."

57 The Xerces Society. *Attracting Native Pollinators*. 2011; Charlotte Rhoades Park and Butterfly Garden website. "Butterfly Species," 2017; Insect Identification for the Casual Observer, website, 2017.

58 Acadia National Park website; Mittelhauser, Glen H., Gregory, Linda L., Rooney, Sally C., and Weber, Jill E. *The Plants of Acadia National Park*, University of Maine Press, 2010.

59 Maine Forest Service, Department of Conservation. *Forest Trees of Maine*. rev., 1995, 17.

60 Acadia National Park website; Maine Forest Service, Department of Conservation. *Forest Trees of Maine*, Polar Bear & Company, 1995 rev.

61 Singer, Gerald. *St. John, Off the Beaten Track*, Sombrero Publishing Co., 2016.

62 Garrison, Bob. *The Last Trail Bandit Guide to the Hiking Trails of St. John, VI*, 2014.

63 Deloach, Ned, and Humann, Paul. *Reef Fish Identification, Caribbean, Florida, Bahamas.* New World Publications, Inc., 2014, Fourth Edition.
64 Kaplan, Eugene. *Coral Reefs, Peterson Field Guides.* Houghton Mifflin, 1982.
65 Snorkel St. John website. 2017.
66 Virgin Islands National Park website. 2017.
67 Collett, Jill, and Bowe, Patrick. *Gardens of the Caribbean.* MacMillan Education Limited. 1988.
68 Hargreaves, Dorothy and Bob. *Tropical Blossoms of the Caribbean.* Ross-Hargreaves. 1980.
69 Honychurch, Penelope N. *Caribbean Wild Plants & Their Uses.* MacMillan Education Limited. 1980, 1986.
70 Lennox, G.W., and Seddon, S.A. *Flowers of the Caribbean.* MacMillan Education Limited. 1978, 1980.
71 Virgin Islands Department of Agriculture, Forestry Division. "Series: Exotic Invasive Species." Department of Agriculture website, 2017.
72 Virgin Islands National Park. Virgin Islands National Park website, 2017.
73 *The Wall Street Journal.* May 5, 2017.
74 Litvaitis, John A., "The Resilient Bobcat," *Northern Woodlands,* Spring 2017, 38.
75 Cornell Lab of Ornithology. *Living Bird,* Winter 2017, 48.
76 Selhub, Eva and Logan, Alan. *Your Brain on Nature.* John Wiley and Sons, Canada, Ltd., 2012.
77 Louv, Richard. *Last Child in the Woods: Saving Our Children from Nature-Deficit Disorder,* Workman Publishing Company, 2005.
78 *Northern Woodlands,* Spring 2017, 28.
79 U.S. Department of Health and Human Services. *National Survey on Drug Use and Health,* 2006.
80 American Psychiatric Association. *Diagnostic and Statistical Manual of Mental Disorders-IV,* American Psychiatric Association, 2000.
81 National Institute of Health website. 2015.
82 U.S. Forest Service website, "Bat Pollination," 2017, 187.
83 Hunter, M.L., Calhoun, A.J.K, and McCullough, M. *Maine Amphibians and Reptiles,* University of Maine Press, 1999.
84 Cornell Lab of Ornithology website. "All About Birds," 2017.
85 Williams, Florence. *The Nature Fix,* W.W. Norton, 2017.
86 Wilson, E.O. *Biophilia,* The President and Fellows of Harvard College, 1986.
87 Beatley, Timothy. *Biophilic Cities,* Island Press, 2010.
88 Louv, Richard. *The Nature Principle,* Algonquin Books of Chapel Hill, 2012.
89 Lyubomirsky, Sonya and Layous, Kristin. "How Do Simple Positive Activities

Increase Well-Being?" *Current Directions in Psychological Science*, in Sage Journals APS, Volume 22, Issue One, 2013.

90 Emmons, Robert and McCullough, Michael. "Counting Blessings Versus Burdens: An Experimental Investigation of Gratitude and Subjective Well-Being in Daily Life," *Journal of Personality and Social Psychology*, June 2010: Volume 98, No. 6, 946-55.

91 Lawrence, Elizabeth, Rogers, Richard, and Wadsworth, Tim. "Happiness and Longevity in the United States," *Social Science Medicine*, 2015, November: 145: 115-119.

92 Gaynor, Michael. "Diet and Depression," *Psychology Today*, website posting October 25, 2014.

93 Lazarus, Arnold. *In the Mind's Eye: The Power of Imagery for Personal Enrichment*, Guilford Press, 1977.

94 Web search "foods that help mood": WebMD.com, September 26, 2017.

95 Web search "foods that help mood": Foodmatters.com, September 26, 2017.

96 Web search: "foods that help mood": Prevention.com, September 26, 2017.

97 Web search: "foods that help mood": EatingWell.com, September 26, 2017.

98 Web search: "foods that help mood": EverydayHealth.com, September 26, 2017.

99 Web search: "foods that help mood": Rodalesorganiclife.com, September 26, 2017.

100 Coon, J. Thompson, Boddy, K., Stein, K., Whear, J., Barton, J., and Depledge, M.H. "Does Participation in Physical Activity in Outdoor Natural Environments Have a Greater Effect on Physical and Mental Well-being than Activity Indoors?" *Environmental Science and Technology*, February 4, 2011.

101 Reynolds, Gretchen. "The Benefits of Exercising Outdoors," *The New York Times*, wellblogs.nytimes.com, February 21, 2013.

102 Paddock, Catherine. "Green Walking Beats the Blues," *Medical News Today*, May 14, 2007.

103 George, Robert. "Just 5 Minutes of Green Exercise Optimal for Good Mental Health," *Medical News Today*. May 4, 2010.

104 Fogel, Alan. "Green Exercise: Exercising Outdoors Has More Benefits than Exercising Indoors," *Psychology Today*, posted February 1, 2010.

105 Peninsula College of Medicine and Dentistry. "Benefits of Outdoor Exercise Confirmed," *ScienceDaily* website, February 5, 2011.